RECHARGED

How my life was enriched by adversity

by

Lin Woolmington

To Sophie & James
with best wishes and love
from Lin xx

First published in Great Britain as a softback original in 2018

Copyright © Lin Woolmington

The moral right of this author has been asserted.

Typeset in Palatino

Design, typesetting and publishing by UK Book Publishing

www.ukbookpublishing.com

ISBN: 978-1-912183-45-6

DEDICATION

To my husband Colin for being my rock. To my daughter Katherine for growing up to be the lovely, amazing person you are. To my grandchildren Jennifer and Jack with thanks for all the delight and fun you give.

My many friends who have been there for me. All who have supported me, especially all the medical staff involved in my rescue, recovery and well being.

---oOo---

LOVE LIFE

by

Lin Woolmington

xxxxxxxxxxxxxxxxxx

Love made my life
Love made me a lover
Love made me a wife
Love made me a mother
~~~
Love made me joyful, jubilant and glad
Love gave me my best times that I ever had
Life made me unhappy, sad and depressed
Life gave me my dark, ugly, unwelcome guest
Love gave me brilliance to see right from wrong
Love gave me tenacity to carry on
Life gave me emotions of sentiment and passion
Life gave me knowledge and wisdom to fashion
Love gave me confidence and comfort to share
Love gave me strength, my burdens to bear
Life gave me courage and guts to face my fear
Love gave me all; the reason I am here.

08.02.2015

---xxXxx---

CONTENTS

---o0o---

CHAPTER I

Cometh the story cometh the book

Nothing had happened to me to be of any literary consequence until my life threatening experience that changed my life completely and forever. I never aspired to be an author but had often heard it said that everyone has a book in them. Wonder what my book would be about? I am sure I would never, ever have foreseen the future that was to be at the heart of my story. When asked what had happened to me I would always truthfully reply, "I had an accident but I don't remember anything about it". Then a dialogue on the following lines would inevitably ensue:

"*What kind of accident?*"

"I said, I don't remember anything about it."

"*Was it a car accident?*"

"No. I said, I don't remember anything about it."

"*But you must have been told.*"

By this time I would start to feel slightly uncomfortable. Why should I tell everyone that I had a life I no longer liked enough to continue living especially when I genuinely had no recollection of the event. Although I regained my composure when I told people how a life threatening experience had enriched my life I felt I needed to develop a coping mechanism to deal with this reoccurring interrogation.

"Wait till the book comes out." These six words were all that was necessary to stop people questioning me. However, their response was invariably "Let me know when?" As a result I was compiling an ever-growing list of email addresses.

My miraculous survival and recovery were featured in a magazine and on television. Many times I was told that I was inspirational. I thought this was incredulous, but I began to believe that it might be worthwhile putting the amazing events in my life into print. If my story was worth telling then I wanted to tell it if it would maybe help someone to understand what clinical depression really felt like. I ventured into public speaking and suggestions to write a book came thick and fast and my enthusiasm for the project grew.

It might be true that everyone has a book in them – but would everyone want to read it? One of my best friends cannot understand anyone being egotistical enough to believe that people would want to read about their life. If she ever reads this one she will know who she is and I love her honesty! I, myself, have never been a very good reader. I guess I had a bad start with the wrong books when I was at school: Silas Marna and Sinbad The Sailor. I know it was the 1950s but surely something more exciting could have been on offer.

I've always enjoyed writing letters and often felt moved to write a poem for specific occasions, so maybe it was possible that I could write a book. At first I doubted that I had enough material for a book, then I realised I had every day of more than 67 years. Gradually memories from all those years entered my head. I enjoyed the sentiment of indulging in my memoirs and before I knew it I started to write them down. However, suddenly a book seemed huge – I could tell my story in half an hour – how was I going to write a hundred pages? Surely any book worth publishing has to have at least a hundred pages. Help!

Every single human life is a true story. Even though human beings have lots of similarities each one has a different aura, and is unique. Whether good or bad, all sorts of things happen to people as they grow up and mature and our lives are continuously changing as we have careers, relationships, accidents and adventures. Many events are similar but there will always be something different to make each one unique, be it the time of year or time of day, the location in the world or age of the person involved. A similar incident or accident can happen to several individual people but the outcome will never be absolutely identical. What can cause one person's life to be shattered forever may give another individual, experiencing a similar happening, a new outlook and deeper understanding of what life is all about.

We are all born into the familiarity of our own surroundings, the feel of our clothes on our skin, the smells that surround us, the warmth of the person holding us. All these sensations provide our comfort and security. They are our 'norm' and for a while they are our world, as far as we know every baby has exactly the same environment.

Babies arrive with no concept of the type of family they have been born into or, indeed, whether they are in the right family. Whether they are rich or poor, what religion their parents follow, if any or whether they have siblings or not. As we grow up and experience life we discover a wide range of lifestyles and types of people. Some will be similar to ours and some will be completely alien. We all have the right to make our own choices as to what to embrace and what to dismiss. All our choices have consequences but we rarely know what those consequences will be as we embark on our adventure of life. We cannot truly know what the future holds but if you have a mind to read on, you will learn what fate had in store for me.

A bad experience can be buried deep within one's subconscious and virtually forgotten. However, there are many triggers such as anniversaries, places, sounds or smells which can become activators and transport us back to the event, causing a traumatic experience to become live again. A bit like a dried seed, which appears dead until the hint of water on the way motivates life to stir within. It is wise, in my opinion, never to leave unfinished business. Confront the issue head on and face the consequences and the sooner the better.

Whatever people experience in their lives there is a story to tell. Who can resist a true story? Don't we all love to hear a true story? Watch people's reactions when you say you have something to tell them. They invariably show interest but tell them it is a *true* story and they will absolutely give you their full attention.

This is my story. It is not a work of fiction or fantasy. It is my own recollection, my own take on my life. There will undoubtedly be different interpretations and opinions of my account, but this is exactly my true version of events as far as my memory allows. I am conscious of the fact that my story may be read by members of my family or close friends as well as strangers. I accept responsibility to reveal my true thoughts and memories. I would rather my family learn the truth during my lifetime than after I have passed away and unable to answer their questions.

---oOo---

CHAPTER II

Pre me

Early in the twentieth century my grandfather Fred White and his wife Evelyn Mary (nee Trevelyan) lived in the Somerset village of West Hatch with their seven children. They had two sons, Toby and Leslie, and five daughters, Christine, Daisy, Doris, Kathleen and Pearl.

Their third daughter was Doris Annie and she had been born on 15 February 1914. The family home where Doris grew up with her six siblings was a very old cottage in a rural location down a country lane. My grandfather, Fred, was a farm labourer while my grandmother, Evelyn Mary, ran her own laundry from the cottage. Between them I would imagine they provided a good, if modest, family life for their children. No doubt their large garden yielded lots of home grown produce for them.

Many years later my sister and I drove to Taunton to visit our cousin Ann who was the daughter of our Aunt Christine, the eldest of our mother's sisters. We all drove out to the location to see our grandparents' old home. The current owners were in the garden so, of course, we engaged them in conversation. They very kindly invited us inside and it was an amazing experience to cross the threshold and enter my grandparents' kitchen. I was standing on ground where my mother would have taken her first steps as a child. The owners showed us the deeds of the property and we learned that our grandmother had been the registered owner of the cottage. She certainly sounds like a lady ahead of her time, running her own business and owning property in that time of the twentieth century. Even so, I wonder what she would have made of my lifestyle today in the twenty-first century?

Doris loved children and, as old photographs show, she was often looking after her younger siblings. They would all go to school together, climbing over the gate of old Farmer Quick's farm and crossing his fields. What an idyllic image that conjures up, seven children scrabbling their way to school, the girls dressed in pinafores and petticoats and the boys in caps and boots. The sun would have been shining, the bees would have been buzzing and the buttercups blooming, as it always does when one reminisces. I visited the school with my mother many years later. We could not enter the building but she showed me a niche in the brick wall where she used to 'sit'; it was just big enough to accommodate her infant bottom. Our visit was just in time, for while there, we learned that the site had been purchased for redevelopment.

After leaving school at the age of fourteen, Doris would have liked to have trained to become a children's nanny. Sadly, as was often the case in those days of large families, a similar expense was not available for all of the children and so like many of her contemporaries, she went into domestic service. Her first employment was locally at Beauchamp House where she stayed for a few years. When she left the job her grateful employers presented her with an inscribed gold watch. Doris really spread her wings when she left her Somerset home to take up a post in the Surrey village of Shalford. The house was called Whitnorth and it fronted onto the main Guildford road. It was quite a distinctive white property, having pillars at the front door straddling the pavement, even as it does today. Also today the property boasts a Grade II listed property blue plaque on its front wall.

Doris Annie White was a very attractive young lady who made friends easily with her work colleagues and enjoyed outings on their precious days off. By the age of nineteen she had met and fallen in love with a young man from a neighbouring village. William Blytheman had good looks, dark curly hair and a zest for life, and he also owned a motorbike. A handsome young man, he was the only son of his devoted parents. The year was 1934 and their fledgling romance blossomed and bloomed during their courtship. They talked about getting married, raising a family and spending the rest of their lives together.

One beautiful day in spring they decided to go for a spin on his motorbike. I actually don't have any idea what the weather was really like on that day but the romantic side of my imagination comes into play when I think of it. The blue sky patched with fluffy clouds as the early seasonal sunshine gently warmed the earth. The fresh scented air, full of promises of the summer to come, just as their burgeoning romance was on the threshold of a new united life. They were together, she rode pillion and felt the comfort of his strong body as she wrapped her arms around him. The wind in their hair, his scarf flapping, they enjoyed the freedom of the open road, free to travel where they wanted. The future was theirs to mould, to plan, to live.

Fate did not step gently that day. Its heavy boot came down and crushed their future in one cruel stamp. One moment they were together, the next she was in an ambulance on her way to hospital. They were cruelly parted and Doris never saw him again, alive or dead. She was unable to attend his funeral and the next two years of her life were spent in hospital far from her home. The injuries she sustained to her back were severe and her badly crushed leg was encased in a plaster cast. A metal cage like frame over her bed shielded her tragically bruised and damaged body from the weight of the blankets.

Doris was bereft and her loss was profound. All the hospital staff were wonderful and did their best but the pain of her grief was intense. All her life's experiences had been good and she had no knowledge of bereavement – even the medical profession of the day seemed to have no true understanding of how to help her deal with what she was going through emotionally. How could anyone provide the comfort she needed? Even her twenty-first birthday was spent in hospital. Without warning her whole life was changed forever, the love of her life was lost, her future was gone. There were so many unanswered questions: What had happened? Why did he die? Would she live? Would she walk again? What about the family she so longed for?

The local newspaper reported the accident:

MOTOR CYCLIST CRASHES INTO CAR

Young Bramley Man Dies from Injuries

"He simply let go of his handlebars and came straight into my car," said Mrs. Stopford Brooke, wife of Mr. Somerset Stopford Brooks, prospective Liberal candidate for the Guildford Division, when giving evidence at an inquest last night at the Royal Surrey County Hospital on the body of William Alfred Frederick Blytheman (22) of Rose Cottage, Eastwood Road, Bramley, who died as a result of injuries sustained when the motor cycle he was riding came into collision, on Tuesday afternoon at Wonersh, with a car driven by Mrs. Brooke.

On the pillion seat of the motor cycle was Miss Doris White (19) of Whitnorth, The Street, Shalford, who sustained fractures to her right leg.

She is detained in the Royal County Hospital, and was last night stated to be comfortable.

The inquest was conducted by Mr. F. W. Smallpiece (Coroner) with a jury, and Mrs. Stopford Brooke was represented by Mr. P.J. Woodhouse (Messeres. Triggs Turner & Co).

"Waved Their Hands"

Addressing the jury, the Coroner said Miss White was not in a condition to give evidence that night, and if the jury thought it necessary for her to be present the enquiry should be adjourned. He understood she could not help them much. All she could say was that they waved their hands to someone on the side of the road.

William Blytheman said his son had ridden the motor cycle only three weeks.

P.C. Rose (Blackheath) said the road at the point of impact was 17 feet wide, and there was a slight bend. The wheels of the car were off the surface of the road. The off-side front mudguard and running board of the car were damaged, and the wheel of the motor cycle was badly buckled, the front tyre burst and both foot rests bent. Adhering to the off-side end of the car door were some human hairs and flesh.

Mrs. Margaret Louise Stopford Brooke, Easteds, Shamley Green said she was driving from Shamley Green to Guildford between 2 and 2.30 p.m. After passing Wonersh crossroads she saw Blytheman on his motor cycle. Her speed was 10 to 15 miles per hour, and the car was on the proper side of the road.

On Wrong Side of the Road

"When I saw him" (Blytheman) continued Mrs. Brooke, "he was about 75 yards away. It was a fairly straight road and I did not think anything about it until he got a bit nearer. He was on the wrong side of the road, and I naturally thought he would pull over, knowing the speed of his own motor cycle, but when he got nearer to me I realised that unless I moved very close over to the nearside of the road he would not be able to pull over to his side. When he was about 20 or 30 yards away from me I started to go onto the grass verge. He simply let go of his handlebars and came straight into me. He seemed to try and pull round."

The Coroner: Have you any idea as to the speed he was travelling? – "I judged that he was going about 35 to 40 miles per hour. He was going very much faster than I was." Mrs. Brooke added that her car was practically stationary when on the grass verge, and directly the car and cycle collided she stopped and got out.

"I stopped a car going from Guildford to Wonersh," proceeded Mrs. Brooke, "and ran towards Dr. Allport's house but a woman said he was out. Eventually someone else sent for a doctor. The injured people were both taken to hospital."

Lying on the Road

The Coroner: Where was the man when you got out of the car? – "He was lying in the middle of the road half beneath the cycle. The girl was on the other side of the road not on the path."

Did you see the driver of the motor cycle or the girl wave their hands? – "No."

Was the girl able to say anything? – "She was perfectly conscious the whole of the time, but only asked if he was alright."

Dr. Francis George Maitland, house surgeon at the hospital, said Blytheman had a compound fracture of the skull over the right eye and severe abrasions to the right side of the face. He died at 4.35 the same day. The cause of death was cerebral compression and laceration of the brain.

The Coroner: What is the condition of the woman? – "She is in a fairly good condition. She has a fracture of the right leg."

The jury expressed sympathy with the relatives of the deceased. With these latter sentiments Mr. Woodhouse associated himself on behalf of Mr. and Mrs. Stopford Brooke.

Among those present at the inquest were Mr. Somerset Stopford Brooke and his father, Mr. S.W.W. Brooke.

The deceased young man was a native of Bramley and was employed at the Guildford Co-operative Society bakery department as a confectioner.

---oOo---

Doris did survive and she did walk again. In fact, one day she walked down the aisle at her wedding when she married her new young man, John Heather. John was also in service, employed as footman to the butler at Oldlands Hall, Uckfield in Sussex and his family home was in the nearby village of Shamley Green. It had been a long hard struggle but it seemed that once again Doris had something to live for. She had found a new love and began to plan for her future once more.

On 17 October 1938 Miss Doris Annie White and Mr John Heather were married in West Hatch church in Somerset. Their first home was a bungalow in New Road in the lovely Surrey village of Wonersh and it was no surprise that they called their new home White Heather. Whilst out walking at the nearby village of Blackheath one day, the newlyweds were dumbfounded to see another property bearing the same name. They removed their home's name sign and replaced it with a new one: Dorijon.

At last it seemed that Doris's life was becoming happy again but, quite early in her married life, a medical problem meant that she was to spend another spell in hospital. She was suffering from ovarian cysts, necessitating the removal of one and a half of her ovaries and her fallopian tubes were to be cut and tied. Such invasive surgery for cysts on the ovaries seems incredible nowadays but no doubt it was standard treatment in the 1930's. What about her dreams of having a family? Sadly, the doctors told her, there would be no babies. Again Doris had to deal with a crushing disappointment.

To lose her first love was so cruel and now to lose hope of ever getting pregnant and having children was unbearably heart-breaking. Fate was still stamping its feet but this time there was an antidote to its cruelty. Doris and John agreed to adopt a baby and were overjoyed when these plans were fulfilled and they became adoptive parents.

No doubt Doris's heart filled with joy as she held a very precious baby, now her daughter, Veronica Mary, in her arms for the first time. The beautiful baby girl soon filled their home with happiness, at last they had a child; and a couple of years later their little daughter had a brother, Geoffrey John, when they adopted a handsome baby boy with long dark eyelashes. The children transformed their existence and filled the void in their lives. The pain of Doris's earlier loss was slowly being replaced by the joy of having her own home with her husband and children. She was living again and enjoying family life at last.

A few years later Doris's sister Daisy and her husband were soon to be leaving their employment in a very large house in the village, so Doris and John applied for the post of live-in help. They were fortunate enough to obtain the position, and they moved their family into the servants' quarters of The Chase in Wonersh. Their bungalow 'Dorijon' was let to provide someone else with a home and also give a welcome boost to their finances. The Heather family was complete and with a better level of security than many had at that time.

The family had several years of a good settled domestic family life before fate struck once more. Doris wasn't feeling well, which was a great worry, not only health-wise but also because of their accommodation arrangements. She and John were very worried about her illness and their family and responsibilities. Finding it difficult to cope, Doris feared something was seriously wrong and sought for an answer from her doctor. What was wrong with her? Was she fatally ill? She could not bear the thought of leaving her husband and young family, knowing full well the pain and difficulty such grief would inflict on them. Another tragedy was unthinkable when things had started to go right for her. Weeks turned into months and still there was no explanation and no end to her worry.

Eventually, her condition was diagnosed. Doris was certainly not terminally ill as she had dreaded, but she was pregnant. Yes, against all the odds, she was pregnant. What must it feel like to have come to terms with the fact that your deepest desire is denied you, so you find an alternative only for it to then become available? I imagine Doris and John would have experienced the full gamut of emotions to this news, which must have turned their lives completely upside down. It might have also caused a few ripples with the medical profession. Maybe the surgeons' skills were not as sharp as their instruments in those days but after an operation, which effectively sterilised her, somehow Doris had healed sufficiently to become pregnant and she was indeed expecting a baby. Her disbelieving doctor told her husband, "You've got some good stuff there, John!"

In the fullness of time on the seventh of September 1945 in the Jarvis Maternity Hospital in Guildford, Doris gave birth to a healthy baby girl. Their new daughter was christened Linda Margaret Heather. Yes, I was that baby.

---oOo---

CHAPTER III

Pre school

For the first three years of my life the Heather family remained living in the servants' quarters of The Chase in Wonersh. Fortunately the owners of the house were a very benevolent family who valued the qualities and intrinsic value of having my parents in residence even with their (now), three children.

I consider the most iconic photograph of me as a child shows me wearing a white organza dress with a blue sash at the waist, sitting on a stone bench on the veranda at the back of the house. An earlier picture of my sister in the same dress shows the skirt full and billowy. I fully endorse passing clothes on to younger siblings and I am amused to note that the hand-me-down dress looks somewhat limp in my photo but I don't mind that at all – it makes me smile. It was at the end of the Second World War but as children of course we weren't aware of any rationing or shortages, we didn't know any different. Obviously my parents had not planned or expected to have another addition to their family, so I guess my arrival must have been quite a shock, not to mention a strain on emotional and financial resources. Another earlier photo of my mother holding me on the same garden seat includes a little black dog, one of two poodles called Bing and Begonia belonging to the owners of the house.

My Dad once told me of a family in his village who could not pay their bills and they were evicted from their house. As a boy he had been very upset by the sight of the contents of their home loaded on a cart before they left the village in the snow one winter. The horror of the workhouse was a real memory to my parents' generation and Dad's understanding was that this family's plight was the result of the man of the house spending too much time and money in the pub to the detriment of his family. A sad lesson in life for post-war austerity, I think there and then Dad must have decided never to give in to the evils of alcohol and I don't think he ever entered a pub. He valued the security of his family home and peace of mind above all else.

Fortunately for us, we were able to stay living at the Chase where my brother and sister and I we were really spoilt with a huge, beautiful garden for our playground. Sweeping lawns went down to the lake and tall, majestic trees added to the splendour as well as providing shade in the summer. Beside the lake near a weeping willow tree was a carved wooden seat. A favourite photograph shows the three of us, all in badly fitting knickers, standing on the bench. I can't help laughing whenever I look at this picture; lycra had definitely not hit the shops then! Nothing and no-one bothered us in the garden. When I think of it now it was like we had our own private park. There was a hidden hazard, however – my poor brother stood in the kitchen one day, screaming in pain and fear as my mother dabbed him all over with a blue bag. He had unfortunately managed to disturb a nest of bees in the garden and they had stung him many times. A blue bag was a block of blue in a muslin bag, made by a company called Reckitt's. Like many other Mums at that time, Mum would use the blue bag in with the white laundry, to make it look even whiter. Whether it really took the pain out of bee stings I don't know but it certainly looked impressive.

Just outside our kitchen was an area like a courtyard. On summer afternoons we would all sit round the table having our tea out there. What a novelty for us to have tea outside. Another favourite family photograph records the scene, complete with a pot of Robinson's jam on the table. The golliwog on the jam label was a replica of the paper golliwog under the lid. These 'gollies' could be collected and sent away to exchange for a metal Robinson's Golliwog badge. Something I did when I was a bit older and had several different golly badges in my collection.

Whether my shoes were buckled or laced I cannot recall but I know I was sitting on the kitchen floor one day, trying to do my shoes up when I realised I was being watched. I looked up to see my Dad's amused expression, full of love, watching me.

Learning to ride a tricycle was wonderful in the safety of the grounds – possibly this is where and when my passion for cycling began. The house had a long gravel drive and a detached garage where the gardener, Mr Higgins, and his family lived in the flat above. One afternoon I was invited to join them for afternoon tea. When asked what I would like to eat, I answered, "Toast with the butter soaked in." I hope I said please!

Many, many years later when my daughter was visiting with her children, my three-year old granddaughter, Jennifer, requested some toast with jam please. It was like hearing an echo from my past and when I produced the iconic photograph of myself aged three in the organza dress and showed it to her she studied it and asked, "Is that me?" When I showed it to Jack, her two year old brother he immediately said, "That's Jennifer."

I was amazed to recently discover that the Chase, now called Wonersh House, was for sale and currently on the market at the reduced price of nine million pounds! After a couple of days wondering whether I should or even could, I girded my loins and popped in to the agent's office. Moments later I popped out again feeling slightly bemused. Having told the friendly, young lady receptionist about my childhood home and explained my interest in the property while admitting that by no means was I a prospective purchaser, she pointed out that, as the property in question was valued at over three million pounds, it would be managed by their international office next door.

So I popped into the neighbouring office where an extremely smart young lady sprang from her desk to shake hands and enquire how she could help. As I got further into my story about the property, two suited gentlemen looked up from their desks to listen in. One of them came forward to join in our conversation and even produced a set of the house details in response to my request as to whether this would be possible. I believe they were genuinely interested in my story and happy to learn some background history about the house. Having got this far I decided to try my luck to see if a discreet viewing would be in order. Unfortunately they felt a visit would not be permissible as the owners lived abroad and the property was securely locked up, but at least I had the glossy brochure to rekindle my memories of the beautiful playground of my youth.

I was three years old when my parents left The Chase and bought a white semi-detached cottage in the village. We all moved into Meadow View Cottage, which was to be our home for more than a decade. Not long after we moved in, the elderly lady who lived on her own in the adjoining cottage went to live with her daughter. My parents bought her vacant cottage and the two properties were knocked into one. The spare staircase was boarded up and became a long storage area. The second staircase remained in use and it had a latch door at the bottom. When I was being corrected for being naughty I was told to sit in the bottom of the stairs (on the naughty step). With the door closed my punishment soon turned into boredom and I would go upstairs and plait the tassels around the bottom of the big armchair in my parents' bedroom. Actually, it was my bedroom too as my cot was in there. This certainly turned out to be fortunate for me on the night that I took a favourite doll and her dummy to bed with me. When my parents retired to bed they were concerned by the strange noise coming from my cot. My mouth was open and lodged in the back of my throat was my doll's red plastic dummy! The dummy was carefully extracted and all was well for a peaceful night.

As was the norm at the time in many homes, heating in Meadow View was provided by an open solid fuel fire in the lounge and a boiler in the kitchen for hot water. I well remember the regular deliveries of coal and anthracite when the coalman, covered in coal dust, would carry sacks full of fuel to our coal shed and shoot the contents out in a cloud of pungent black dust. Sometimes our fuel didn't seem to last as long as it should so I was told to keep count of the number of sacks delivered to make sure we were not short changed. Upstairs heating was provided by electric or oil fires in the bedrooms. I remember the pattern made on the ceiling by the holes in the top of the portable oil heater. I also remember the exquisite patterns of frost on the windowpanes on winter mornings.

A year or two after we moved into Meadow View, the north end of the house was surrounded in scaffolding while a bathroom was added to the building with a further bedroom above it. I was to have my own bedroom at last. My room was at the back of the house and I loved the view from the window. I could see straight into the back garden and the green hill beyond, then the woods, topped by a stone-built tower on the skyline. It was magical.

Although he had no formal training Dad proved to be very capable at putting his hand to most jobs that needed to be done to our new home. One day I watched in fascination as he mixed sand and cement with water using a large shovel and he then laid a new concrete path at the back of the house. I was probably about five years old at the time and I pressed my hand into the wet cement and wrote my name in the path. About fifty years later I was out on my bike one summer when I cycled past the house. A further extension had since been added, the garden wall had been replaced by a high hedge and the ramshackle garage had been improved somewhat, but to me it was still unmistakably my old home. An elderly couple were standing at the gate saying goodbye to some visitors, I looked as I passed and looked back again, over my shoulder. Their visitors gone, the couple at the gate waved to me – they must have thought I knew them, or maybe they knew me. I pedalled a few more yards, then stopped. Seize the moment, I thought. I dismounted, turned my bike round and rode over to the gate. The couple were charming and when I told them I grew up in Meadow View to my surprise they asked if my name was Heather! "Yes," I said, "that was my surname." I accepted their invitation into the house feeling as if I was in a dream of magical nostalgia. I entered the room where, after our meal, we had discovered a puppy in a box under the table. It seemed a much smaller room than I remembered but it was, without doubt, the very room. With the passing years the house had been much modified, the old staircase had been reinstated and it wasn't easy to recognise very much. Nevertheless, it was wonderful to revisit my childhood home and a joy to see my handprint still there in the cement path.

Meadow View had proved to be a lovely home. I loved the house, the garden and all my friends and memories in the attractive village of Wonersh.

My parents had friends in Guildford called Dick and Dorothy, who did not have a bathroom in their house, they did, however, to my fascination, have a daughter who was a professional ice skater in Tom Arnold's Holliday on Ice. This was a popular show at the time. Sometimes when they visited, Dorothy was offered the opportunity to enjoy the luxury of soaking in a lovely hot bath. After one such occasion there was a bit of a panic when Dorothy's engagement ring, which she had removed before bathing, went missing. Oh dear, what a to-do, Dorothy was not happy, and Mum felt terrible that the ring was lost in our house. The loss of the ring was often spoken about, we were all to keep our eyes peeled and hope it could be found. After some time, emotions calmed down and Dorothy visited again and enjoyed another bath. This time she emerged from the bathroom sheepishly, looking somewhat embarrassed. As she had taken the cap off her tin of talcum powder she discovered her ring where she had carefully placed it, on the neck of the tin!

My parents' friends were members of the All Nations Club, which was based in Guildford at the time. The Club often held social events and sometimes I would attend the Club's dances at Trinity Church Hall in Guildford, with the friends. These were very friendly affairs and the dances were very easy. Some, such as the Paul Jones, were progressive, so after every sequence of steps the dancers moved on and danced with the next partner. It was interesting to dance with someone from Japan then someone from Africa, or maybe a Frenchman or an American; they literally were from all nations.

The same friends lived in a house in St Joseph's Road in Guildford, situated right opposite the now vanished Guildford City football ground. Whenever there was a home football match many men would arrive on their bicycles and pay three pence each to park their bikes in the garden. When I was a bit older and my parents' friends were away on holiday, a friend and I were allowed to be parking attendants and collect the money for pocket money.

Our house in Wonersh was set back from the road by an area of common, the front garden had a walled boundary, the big back garden had two apple trees and a Victoria plum tree, and the view from the back of the house was the grassy hill with woodland beyond and a stone-built tower at the top. We never had to buy apples; whenever we wanted one we just picked it from the tree. One of the trees produced cooking apples while the other produced Russett eating apples. When the fruit was ready I remember my brother and I harvesting them and placing the best ones on flat wooden trays. Dad would then store them in the loft, ready for use during the winter. Dad was a keen kitchen gardener, growing many of the vegetables that made up a large part of our diet. I often lifted the potatoes into a bucket as Dad dug along the row, turning over a spit of soil to reveal the tubers snuggled in the earth. One frosty day while I was cutting Brussels sprouts from the stalk, I managed to slice my little finger as well. As she tended to my wound my Mum put her little finger next to mine and told me that when I was born she compared our little fingers and marvelled at how similar they were.

Our front garden at Meadow View was well stocked with plants; I remember fuchsias, irises and lupins in the borders and yellow roses round the porch at the front door. It was possible to walk all the way round the house and at one side there were straight concrete walls up to the chimney, perfect for playing two-ball. I adored this game of keeping two balls going, alternately throwing them at the wall and catching them. Many happy hours were spent perfecting the skill and learning all the intricate moves to make the game more interesting. The concrete paths provided perfect areas for skipping, another favourite pastime. I could skip equally well forward and backwards and do 'bumps' (turning the rope twice while jumping once). How satisfying to hear the swish of the rope when the speed doubled.

The front room or sitting room had a large black wooden beam across the ceiling and an inglenook fireplace. Each of the chimneys on either side had a wooden seat. It was brilliant in the winter to sit in a chimney corner seat and feel the warmth of the open fire in the grate. It was also lovely to sit by the fire and listen to the wireless.

"When the music stops Daphne Oxenford will be here to speak to you." Ding de dong, ding de dong, ding de dong, ding de dong, diinggg went the musical jingle, then Daphne would speak to me: "Are you sitting comfortably? Then I'll begin."

It is the early 1950s, and I am a young child, sitting on a pouffe by the open fire in the sitting room at a quarter to two in the afternoon. With my ear close to the bakelite wireless I am listening to 'Listen with Mother' on the Home Service. Daphne Oxenford is the presenter and is now saying that she is going to tell me a story. All this I can remember very clearly but I cannot remember even one of the many stories she told. Nevertheless, it is a good heart-warming memory, evoking all the senses of home and security, very much a part of my early childhood.

A large wooden door in the sitting room opened into a cupboard in the wall, big enough to walk into and, sometimes, hide in. It was a wonderful storage area for all our toys and games.

Before the bathroom was added to the house our weekly bath night involved the grey tin bath being taken down from its hook on an outside back wall, brought into the lounge in front of the fire and filled with kettles and saucepans of hot water. Mmm, am I really old enough to remember baths by an open fire? Yes, I am! Sometimes there was an added treat. If she hadn't made my bed up, Mum would change the sheets and make it 'with me in it'! When the bottom sheet was in place I would lie on the bed and have the top sheet thrown over me like a billowing tent and I'd wriggle and giggle as the bed was 'made with me in it'. I love this childhood memory, one of many of our time at Meadow View.

There were occasional childhood ailments to keep me home from school. Whilst it was horrid to be really ill with mumps, measles, or bronchitis, which I was prone to suffer from in winter, feeling poorly with a bad cold was almost to be enjoyed. A day in bed reading and daydreaming then hearing the familiar creak of the stairs as Mum approached with warm drinks and meals on a tray to aid recovery. Mmm, I must say I was a fortunate patient.

I don't think a good smack did my siblings or me any harm and although we were all subject to the discipline of the day and the resulting tears and pain, they now seem insignificant moments, far outweighed by good memories of parental love.

There was something like a fire hydrant just inside the garden wall that made a wonderful 'step' for me to climb up and join my older brother and sister and often several friends, sitting on the wall. The grass on the common area beyond our garden wall would grow pretty high in the summer. I loved the time when it was cut down by the Council, the smell of newly cut grass would fill the air and it meant I could play dive bombing with my friends. We would pile the hay up high into a big mounds and dive into the middle of it.

On the other side of the road from our house was a ditch and tall hedge, then another row of houses. The Bowbrick family lived in the house on the corner; they owned the local dairy and our milk was delivered in grey metal milk churns on their lorry. The required amount was ladled out into our own container.

Two of my friends also lived in the houses across the road. I remember playing in one friend's garden one summer and getting very messy making mud pies. My very first night away from home was spent staying with the other friend. I recall the occasion when I was having tea with them. Everyone seated round the table, my friend and I, her parents and her maiden aunt. Several families I knew had a maiden aunt; they were often ladies who had lost their sweethearts in the war and never married. My Dad's youngest sister Nellie was my own maiden aunt.

Just beyond our garden gate there was a slope where the common area was a little higher than our pathway. It was covered in snow one winter when Mum and I set out to walk to the bus stop. Disaster struck when Mum slipped on the slope and fell in the snow. I wonder now just how the ambulance arrived with no mobile phone to instantly summon help, but arrive it did. I watched in impressed concern as my mother was wrapped in red woollen blankets and carried into the vehicle on a stretcher. Poor Mum had broken her ankle of her 'good' leg. On the plus side, we got to keep the red hospital blankets with black stripes at one end and green blanket stitch at the edges. They became favourite extra bed coverings on winter nights and lasted for many years.

---oOo---

CHAPTER IV

Growing up in the village

The Second World War ended four months before I was born in 1945. The fear of war was over but the memory still lingered and there were reminders of that terrible time even in my early childhood. As a very young child I recall seeing a comic with references to Hitler as a swine and cartoon drawings of him depicted as a pig. I also remember my Mum wearing a blouse that was very soft and finely woven; she said it was made out of parachute silk from the war. There were quite a number of ex-prisoners of war who stayed in England and some were working on the land in the nearby village of Shamley Green in Surrey. When two of them were looking for accommodation they came to Meadow View and lodged with us. Karol Ludwick Choykawski was a Polish man and Egan Brent was a German. My parents had no prejudices. Egan was a very kind, dark haired young man. One day he gave me a white toy dog with a bright red plastic collar with a buckle. Like one of my teddy bears, it was stuffed with straw, which found its way through the paws after much play and its collar doubled as a bracelet for me. There was an incident one day when Egan had been out drinking and was ill when he returned. Very shortly after this he moved away and we never saw him again. This incident left a lasting impression in my immature mind: how bad the consequences could be from drinking too much alcohol.

Karol was an older man, also kind and talented at woodwork and painting. Being a catholic he always received a letter at Easter time enclosing a wafer of communion bread from his sister Ann in Poland. How hard it must have been for these two men to find themselves in a foreign country looking for a home and employment. I like to think their families would have been comforted by the fact that they had good accommodation with an English family. Karol would often take me to Holland's shop in the village and say to Eileen "I want some sweets for my sweet". One day he took me to the pictures to see The Hunchback of Notre Dame. Apart from Quasimodo swinging on the bell ropes and capturing a pretty young woman, I just remember squalid scenes of the low life in Paris. I now question whether it was a suitable film for me at such a young age but I don't believe it did me any harm.

There used to be a second-hand bookshop in Guildford called Thorpe's. It was a 'must' for any trip to town. I certainly wasn't a bookworm but something about this rambling building, which had once been a cinema, fascinated me. It must have housed thousands of second-hand books; they filled all the shelves on the walls from floor to ceiling and were stacked in piles on every step of the staircase. Karol once took me to Thorpe's and asked for a copy of Quo Vadis? (Whither Goest Thou?) by Henryk Sienkiewicz. The book was produced and Karol bought it. He later gave it to me and he had written in the flyleaf: *This book I gift to Linda Heather for memory in 1954 February. K L Choykawski.* I started to read it once but it was harder going than Silas Marner or Sinbad the Sailor! I kept the book and years later in 2007 (after Karol had passed away) when we took a short holiday break to Krakow in Poland I put a photograph inside the cover of the book and took it with me. Krakow was Karol's home town and the photo was of my Dad, my brother, me and Karol in the garden of Meadow View, with our dog, Bambi. I had no idea whether any of Karol's family still lived in Krakow but I felt that in some way he would be nearer his family if I took the book with me. It seemed the right thing to do. Karol kept in touch with us until he died but he left our home when he married an English lady called Mary.

For me, growing up in the 1950s life had a reassuring unhurried routine. Shops were closed on Sundays and Wednesday afternoons – that was always half-day early closing. Sunday lunch was always a roast meal with gravy and a pudding to follow, all enjoyed with Family Favourites on the radio. This was a musical request programme for British Forces serving overseas. Monday was laundry day and our main meal was cold meat from the previous day's roast. Friday's meal was usually fish.

Like any other village, Wonersh had its annual events and fair share of characters. The annual Summer Fete on the village green was a great experience. One year my Mum made some toffee apples; they were a great hit and orders for more were sent up to our house. They were the best toffee apples I've ever tasted. Another year an unusual visitor aroused great interest. The Chase, where we used to live, was now called Wonersh House and was owned by an Arab Sheik. He graced our village fete with his presence, wearing his white flowing robes. All this was reported, with pictures, in the Surrey Advertiser. At the 1953 fete I joined all the other children of the village queuing up to be presented with our Coronation Mugs to mark the coronation of Queen Elizabeth II.

There was a French lady who could often be seen walking round the village with her Pekingese dog called Nonny. Maybe she had lost her sweetheart in the war like so many other spinsters of the time. I loved to stop and stroke her lovely little canine creature with its beautiful tail curled up on its back. For years I believed Pekingese were called Nonny dogs. Sometimes late in the evening the sound of hobnail boots could be heard in the distance, accompanied by the sound of singing as a somewhat inebriated resident wandered back from a pub in Guildford, past our house, to his home at the end of the village. My Mum would say, "There goes ol' Frank Sinatra." Of course, I believed that was his real name. His boots were Army boots; I bet he'd have some stories to tell.

A rare sight and sound in the village was the cry of the rag and bone man as he trundled along the road with his horse-drawn cart. No doubt Steptoe and Son on the television owed much of its success to living memory. I doubt today's generation would appreciate it in the same way.

Very often, early on a Sunday afternoon, an elderly man would ride his bike past our house and take the first right hand turning up Blackheath Lane. At the top of the hill was Blackheath village and the cemetery where he would lay the flowers he had carefully carried whilst cycling along. There was no florist in the village so I guess he grew the flowers in his garden. His name was Mr Hales. Mum said he always took the flowers and visited the grave of his wife. Indeed, there were many times after Sunday school when we would walk up the track across the road from the cricket green to Blackheath and wander round the cemetery reading the gravestones to work out how old people were when they died. I often remember being emotionally moved to see the shape of a man kneeling on the ground beside a grave. The grave was just inside the cemetery gate on the left and the man was Mr Hales.

Mr Hales lived further along the common in the last house before the gateway to the fields. When all the hay in the field had been harvested it was piled high into a huge haystack in the shape of a house, the like of which I have since only ever seen in pictures. One particular summer day I found myself with a few friends and some older children playing in and on the haystack. I'm not sure how I got to the top of it but I remember sliding down it many times. It was the best fun ever; the more we climbed and slid, the more fun it became as the haystack began to fall apart, leaving hollow areas, just right for diving into. Who knows how many hours we spent at play completely unobserved by an adult. There is no doubt we would have been in big trouble had we been caught. It might well have even been a case for the local policeman. He had paid us a visit once about an incident over some garden cloches, I think my brother was questioned! It's interesting that we never heard of any trouble over the wrecked haystack – at least, I didn't.

We had a lovely big grey rabbit called Bimbo who lived in a large hutch at the back of the house. Our big black cat was called Whiskey, and she had lovely soft fur. During a tremendous storm I recall sitting in our lounge with Whiskey snuggled on my lap as great flashes of lightning blazed into the room and booming rumbles of thunder rolled around. It seemed as if Whiskey and I kept each other safe and comfortable during the storm.

I was very excited one day when Mum and I came back from the pet shop in Guildford with a guinea pig. White hair grew in rosettes all over her body; she was an Abyssinian guinea pig, I called her Topsy and enjoyed looking after her. Shortly after getting Topsy I was holding her in my hands when I thought something was amiss. I was a bit scared and called my Mum in alarm – what had happened to my guinea pig? I held a mass of something wet as well as Topsy. It transpired that we had purchased a pregnant guinea pig and she had given birth to her babies in my hand. Wow! We found homes for most of the babies but kept one as company for Topsy. When more guinea pigs arrived, however, we realised we had mistakenly kept a male. This time we kept the runt of the litter; a little black bundle with only one eye – I called him Nelson and he did not share his home with Topsy.

There was another surprise in store one day for my brother and sister and me. When we had all finished our tea and while we were still sitting round the table Mum said there was something for us under the table. What on earth could it be, under the table? Three excited children crouched down and peered into the gloom. I remember seeing a cardboard box similar to the one our groceries arrived in every week.

Like everyone else's Mum at the time mine had a notebook in which orders for our weekly supplies were written. The order book would be taken to the shop and returned with our grocery delivery. I recall that salt was supplied in a paper-wrapped block and I remember sitting at the kitchen table scraping the big white wedge of salt with a knife so Mum could use it for cooking or to fill our salt cellar.

Something seemed to be moving in this box; was it alive? Yes, it was and the cutest little puppy dog looked up at us. She was brown and black, just an adorable puppy, and we called her Bambi. For many years Bambi brought great joy to our lives. How I loved walking through the fields and woods with her after school. She gave me my introduction to the countryside with all its smells, plants, sounds and blissful solitude. I am surprised that I don't want a dog in my adult life, but I don't. Today's society demands that dog owners 'poop scoop'. I'm sorry but I don't think I could lift dog poo, even in a poly bag, without retching, and I'm not prepared to find out.

The best of summer pastimes was walking Bambi along the common to the fields that flanked the village. There were many routes to choose. One path ran at the foot of the field towards Bramley and came out to the road by Wonersh Hollow. This was a short, super, sweeping hill, great for freewheeling down on a bicycle, curving round to the left and over the river before having to pedal again. Taking this path on a walk with Dad one day in late summer when I was very young and riding on his shoulders, from my vantage point, I spotted ripe fruit on a peach tree virtually hanging over the garden wall. Dad slowed his pace to a standstill and leaned against the wall. I felt conscious that I shouldn't really but I stretched out and held the pinky golden fruit in my hand. With my father's silent permission I tugged, and a peach was mine – my first delicious taste of scrumping!

The hills and woods behind Meadow View were wonderful areas for adventures with friends. There were chestnuts to gather in autumn – how sweet they were when the brown and white peel was broken open with my teeth and then the white skin peeled away to reveal the juicy, crunchy chestnut. Mmm, so much better to be eaten before it was fully ripe and the dry skin so difficult to remove. Stomping through the grass and brambles we often made our way through the wooded area to the tower at the top of the hill. To my young fertile imagination this area was a bit remote, magical and slightly scary. I didn't venture there on my own – one never knew what or who could be hiding in the tower. We had to climb over a fence at the edge of the wood to reach the tower and if I remember correctly, there was a sign in the woods saying 'Trespassers will be prosecuted'. Although we didn't fully understand what prosecuted meant we always crept into the tower with great secrecy. The tall stone building felt cold and damp and somehow forbidden. Having dared to enter and creep around it was wonderful to safely run out again into the sunlight.

In winter when the village was deep in snow, the hill with the tower on top provided a terrific run for sledging. Most of the juvenile inhabitants and a few adults would drag their toboggans or carry their tea trays to the top and slide down on them in the snow. It was a wonderful sport and all the colourful woolly hats and coats made it a winter wonderland scene. My bedroom was at the back of the house so I had a wonderful view. In all weathers, throughout the seasons, I could see the hill, the woods and the tower.

A fascinating outing with my Dad was a visit to the Guildford cattle market. We would mingle with livestock dealers as they inspected cattle and sheep corralled in large metal pens. I well remember the live poultry auctions where chickens were held upside down by their feet, their wings falling open and their loud squawking at the indignity of it all.

A trip to Guildford with Mum would often include a visit to Sainsbury's in the High Street. Supermarkets had not been heard of and this grocery and provisions store seemed to have miles of counters with lots of assistants to serve you. There were marble counters for the dairy products section. Here the assistants, usually female, wore white coats and hairnets. They would slice off a portion of butter, deftly shape it with wooden butter pats before placing it on the scales to determine weight and price then wrap it in greaseproof paper for the customer. Each commodity had its own section and was purchased separately in that section.

I often went on shopping errands for my Mum and a visit to the village shops meant a walk down the common then across the road. On the common was a big tree trunk; it was all that remained of a once huge, proud tree. It was my delight to go and play for hours with friends on 'the log'. The local sweetshop was called Holland's and was run by an elderly lady called Mrs Holland with her daughter and son-in-law, Mr and Mrs Butt. My mother still referred to Mrs Butt by her maiden name, Eileen Holland. From time to time travelling businessmen would call into Holland's shop and ask if they knew of anywhere they could find accommodation in the village. So it was that we had occasional lodgers. Despite the extra work, Mum was always happy cooking and looking after people and of course it helped financially. One such visitor stayed with us several times and liked the location so much he once brought his wife to visit us. Another lodger was a young man called John Wesley Bailey; I guess his parents were members of the Wesleyan Chapel. He had a motorcycle and I can remember him riding alongside me as I cycled to school, his left hand on my back so I was effectively being pushed along without having to pedal. No way could I imagine that happening today, I'm glad I grew up in the 1950s.

Another shop in the village was Faulkner's, the newsagents and general store. Getting up early to deliver newspapers had its rewards: earning some pocket money. When I was about eight or nine years old, there was a vacancy so I went to see Mr Faulkner who said he would drive me round the delivery route in his van. Much to Mum's astonishment, I went straight out early one morning without having my hair plaited, something I would not normally do. Mr Faulkner was taking me out in his van to show me the route of my proposed paper round. I obviously valued employment above appearance and was chuffed when I was given the job of being papergirl for Shamley Green. I had to start out really early in the morning, my bicycle panniers bulging with newspapers, and ride up two hills before I started my deliveries. The pleasure of this employment was largely dependent on the weather. I remember delivering in summer and winter so I must have done it for at least a year.

A highlight of the school holiday calendar was potato picking in the summer. Joining several friends in a local farmer's dusty or muddy field we would spend the day practically bent double gathering potatoes in return for pocket money. This occupation was also dependent on fine weather so when it rained and we just sheltered in the barn we did not get paid.

Most of my school holidays involved a journey on the Royal Blue coach to Taunton in Somerset with my Mum and my brother and sister, to stay with my maternal grandmother, Evelyn Mary. If nothing else these trips increased my geographical knowledge of England; the coach travelled through Hartley Witney, Salisbury, Kingsworthy and Abbotsworthy, Yeovil and Ilminster. At Bournemouth the driver would pull into the coach station and we would have a short time to 'stretch our legs' and admire the flower borders in a nearby park before boarding another coach for the remainder of the journey. I never saw and was never aware of our luggage being transferred to another coach but it was always there in the hold on our arrival in Taunton.

One of these coach journeys in the early 1950s gave me my first experience of flooding. Some rural roads in the West Country were under water; only the tops of field gateposts were visible above the water level as were the tops of hedges. Carefully and slowly our coach managed to get through and complete our journey.

My grandmother lived on her own as my grandfather had passed away and her house was within walking distance of Taunton town in the cul-de-sac called Greenway Avenue. There were residential roads right and left off the avenue but at the end was a large green area with a children's playground. What a delight! I don't imagine my grandmother thought about us when she moved into No 42, but I thought it was great, very opportune of her to live so near swings, seesaws and roundabouts. Diagonally across the green was a footbridge over the railway line then a footpath leading into the town. Grandma referred to this bridge as forty-steps, often saying she was 'going over forty-steps'. I can't believe we never counted the steps to see if Grandma was right, but strangely I don't remember how many there actually were. Somewhere beyond the steps we could walk to a park area with a river and a weir; this was quite an adventure – well out of sight of Grandma's house. In later years when my sister was older, she would holiday with her friend at Grandma's house. That seemed really grown up to stay away from home with a friend and no parents!

When my grandmother became seriously ill my Mum made the coach journey to Taunton on her own and left Dad in charge of the three of us. I don't recall any problems during the weeks Mum was away so Dad must have coped very well to feed and clothe us without the convenience of a freezer or washing machine, or television to entertain us. Most little girls with long hair in those days would wear it in pigtails and I was no exception. Poor Dad did struggle with plaiting my hair but I know he did his best.

I think I was about ten years old when I joined the cast of the Pageant of Wonersh. It was produced and directed by an enterprising young man in the village, to portray the history of Wonersh. His name was Peter Osborne and he lived in one of the lovely houses overlooking the village green; I think he may have worked for the BBC. A large cast was gathered from the village residents, including lots of children. A friend and I were cast as flower sellers. I was very glad we did not have any words to learn. Being dressed up as a flower girl wasn't something I felt very comfortable with – nothing against flower sellers, I just didn't like being in costume. In fact, I didn't really enjoy acting very much at all; I would rather have been making the costumes or sitting in the audience. At least I can say I was involved in the Pageant of Wonersh and I do have a photograph of the cast to prove it.

Once, and only once, I attended the Brownies. I thought it would be good, lots of activities with friends, learning lots of things and getting to go away to camp in the summer. Well, somehow I didn't take to their games or their songs – singing about "going down the garden to eat worms" wasn't my idea of fun. To be honest I thought they were all a little mad. I'm sorry about that because I do believe in the good of clubs like the Brownies, Cubs, Guides and Scouts but I think I was looking for something with more meaning at that time in my life so it was not for me. A friend of mine used to go to the St John's Ambulance Brigade so I went along to that and enrolled as a cadet. It meant a bus trip to Guildford followed by quite a long walk to their headquarters but it was much more to my liking. We learnt about first aid, how to help people and how to make beds properly with 'hospital corners' (I still do these when tucking the sheets in). I even liked the cadet uniform, a short sleeved cotton dress in pale grey denim and ruffled white elasticated cuffs above the elbow;

just a bit like a nurse. While I was in the St John's Cadets we had an inspection by royalty. The tallest cadet (me) was the marker at the corner while all the others had to fall in line and take up their positions in the parade ground. This event took place at Woodbridge Road in Guildford and we were inspected by the Queen's sister, Her Royal Highness Princess Margaret.

My attendance at the Guildford St John's Ambulance Centre also gave me a somewhat unwanted but realistic introduction to the adult world. During my walk from the bus station to the cadet centre one week I was aware of a car parked ahead of me and as I passed it the driver moved slowly forward and then parked again. This performance was repeated until I reached the Centre. I told my parents and Dad said that in future he would meet me at the bus stop when I came home. The following week the same car shadowed my walk again but this time it was still there when I walked back to the bus station. I knew I was safe when my Dad was there to meet me at the village bus stop, but so was the car. The driver had followed the bus all the way. Fortunately that episode ended that night and I continued attending the St John's Cadets and my Dad always met me at the bus stop.

One Christmas morning I had one of the best surprises of my life. I was over the moon when I saw my Christmas present – a brand new bike. It was made by Bluemels and had a pale blue frame with bright shiny spokes in the wheels. Cycling to school was good and riding home with friends was even better. At the point where one friend and I should have said goodbye and gone off in different directions to our homes, we would stop for a chat. That chat would often last for an hour or more – whatever we found to talk about for so long is now a mystery to me.

Weekends and summer evenings were great for cycle rides with another school friend. We often rode in the Godalming area. Little did I know that one day that would be where I was to live. We would often pack sandwiches for lunch and go out for the day. It was long before mobile phones were available but I don't think our Mums worried about us; anyway we always turned up back at home in time for tea. As we didn't have a television I often cycled over to a friend who lived in Shalford, to watch The Goon Show on her telly. One evening I was a bit late and it was getting dark before I left my friend's house. I had no lights on my bike and wondered whether I would have the disgrace and bad luck to be stopped by a policeman – I knew it was against the law to ride without lights after dark. To take my mind off the prospect of being accosted by the law, I talked to an imaginary passenger on the back of my bike. I gave a running commentary on the entire journey, mentioning every turning, every gateway and landmark; "We're nearly there," "not far now". At last my home was in sight, I pedalled as fast as I could and breathed a huge sigh of relief when I dismounted and pushed my bike through our garden gate. I was safely home and not a policeman in sight.

In June 1960 my sister got married and her wedding reception was held in the garden at Meadow View. It was a lovely sunny day and as photographs show, it was a very happy occasion.

Soon after this we moved to a smaller three bedroomed semi-detached house in the nearby village of Shalford. The move made sense for practical reasons as our house was quite large for my parents to maintain, but I for one was not happy about it. I stayed in my bedroom until the last possible moment and was very reluctant to leave my beloved Meadow View.

---oOo---

CHAPTER V

School days

In the first week of September in 1950, at the age of five, I became a pupil at the Infants' School in the neighbouring village of Shalford. My first day at school started with a ride on the school bus with the other boys and girls in the village. I envied the children who arrived by travelling in a little seat on the back of their Mum's bike but understood that my Mum did not ride a bike. My brother and sister and I all started our education in the same infants' school, but by the time it was my turn they had moved up to the Primary School so I hardly remember being at school with them. It was good that friends I had made locally were now my school friends. We could play together at school as well as after school and at weekends. Fortunately we still had a good size garden, nothing like the Chase, but plenty of room for safely playing with friends.

I remember my Mum gathering my brother and sister and I together after school one day. I was about six, my brother about nine and my sister about eleven and Mum said she had something to tell us. She said that someone at school had said to my sister "Mrs Heather isn't your real mother". And she explained that my brother and sister were adopted. I think they may have already known, there didn't seem to be any upset over the news or maybe we were too young to understand exactly what adoption meant. I just knew I had a brother and sister so why should it make any difference to me how they had arrived? When Mum told me that they were special and they were chosen, I imagine she didn't want me to think of my siblings as being any less loved than I was. I tried to understand what she told me but began to wonder why I wasn't special and chosen. Later I began to wonder how my brother and sister viewed my presence now that they had to share their parents' love and attention with a third party.

At the age of eight I moved up to Shalford Primary School, which was conveniently situated next to the Infants'. Transport to school was still via the school bus and I remember waiting in the bus shelter just across the common in front of our house and climbing on with other children to join the others already on board. There was something very friendly about the school bus. No rules and regulations and no squabbling, bragging or fighting. We all just climbed aboard and were taken to school. One memorable ride home, however, ended when I was unceremoniously shoved from behind just as I stepped off the bus. Tears pricked my eyes as I flinched and yelled whilst lying in a ditch full of stinging nettles. One of the boys on the bus had decided it would be fun to push one of the girls into the ditch. I'll never know if my experience was just by chance or had I been specially singled out for this treatment? Had it happened today he would most likely be reported for bullying, but then it was just something school kids did and it was all but forgotten. Although I do still remember it, at the time it gave me a painful nettle rash whereas now it just gives me a good laugh.

The village of Shalford was fortunate enough to boast the location of an authentic, historic, old flour mill and one day we were all marched about half a mile down the road to visit the mill. I remember climbing old wooden stairs, seeing the huge mill wheels and grinding stones. The mill has an amazing history and today it is owned by the National Trust who organise hands-on craft activity days for children. I love the idea that one day, in the not too distant future, I will hopefully take my grandchildren on a visit to explore Shalford Mill.

We were also lucky enough to have another out of school activity. The whole class crossed the road outside the school and walked along a path over the railway bridge and into a field between the railway line and the river. There were several shallow narrow ditches criss-crossing the field and our teacher divided the area into plots for us to inspect. Our mission was to conduct an ordnance survey of the field and find out what plants and wildlife inhabited it.

There was another occasion when I recall walking down the village in a 'crocodile' with my fellow pupils. Her Majesty The Queen and The Duke of Edinburgh were coming to Shalford! We were all lined up on the pavement to await the drive past of the royal car. Fortunately the weather was fine for this auspicious occasion, as the royal couple rode in a black, open-top vehicle so we could clearly see the recently crowned Queen and her husband waving to us all. We all cheered and waved back. I bet I wasn't the only one who thought the Queen actually looked at her. It truly was a day to remember.

Out of the back gate at the bottom of the school playground and across the road was an area of land, half of which was laid out for each pupil to have a little plot of garden. Here we could plant our own seeds and watch flowers and vegetables grow. I do remember marvelling at anything that materialised in my plot; unfortunately I was not blessed with green fingers and even to this day I do not have success with growing flowers or keeping pot plants alive. I wouldn't call it a lawn but the other half of this land was a grassy area where we had some of our sports events. I didn't exactly enjoy sports but possibly because I had the longest legs, I was the best at the high jump in my class and wasn't too bad at the long jump either.

"The time you have just spent in the playground has now passed; you will never have that time again." I was about ten years old when

I heard my primary school headmaster address the class one day when we returned to the classroom at the end of playtime. It is a pity he has now passed away too – I can never tell him that his words have certainly not been forgotten by me, they have often been quoted by me and now have been written by me, in a chapter of my book. He was very smart and upright, almost with a military bearing, I've always admired good posture and he had very tidy dark, wavy hair. His arrival was heralded by the sharp click of his shoes as he strode across the playground or classroom. My primary school headmaster was a man of discipline and I liked him even though he once referred to me as a clucking hen when I was talking in class. ("No surprise there," I hear some friends mutter).

I enjoyed my school days and I even loved school dinners, especially butterscotch tart. I also think my generation were the lucky ones to have free school milk. Along with the doses of Radio Malt, which I loved, and Scott's Emulsion, which I did not, that my Mum spooned out to each of us every day, we had a good healthy start in life. Whilst at primary school we all had to walk in a 'crocodile' to the village hall where lunch was served. I have vivid memories of two lunchtime events in this hall. Firstly, the day when complete silence followed a sudden loud bang. Members of staff ate at a table on the stage and one teacher had banged the saltcellar on the table to try and unblock it. I think he was even shocked by the volume of noise his action caused.

Secondly, when we were all lined up with our plates queuing for lunch one day, we noticed a tiny circle of bright sunlight coming through a knot-hole in the timber hall wall and jostled each other to focus the light on our own plate. Whether this triggered something in one boy's mind I don't know but he promptly recited a rather rude rhyme, which for some inexplicable reason I have never forgotten: "Fart is a mechanical eruption, it comes from the mountain of bum, passes through the valley of arseholes and comes out with a musical hum!" Very rude, typical schoolboy humour and it still makes me giggle.

Our journey to the village hall involved crossing the railway line via a wooden footbridge. Sometimes our crossing coincided with a steam train passing underneath or stopping for water. When this was the case, we would squeal excitedly, running across the bridge to dodge the thick black smoke billowing from the train engine's funnel. Watching the driver refill the water tank from a large rubber hose hanging from a framework by the track, reminded me of a huge elephant's trunk swaying around squirting water everywhere. When the steam whistle sounded the train would steam out of the station and chug away out of sight; one direction went to Guildford and the other to Dorking.

After crossing the railway we walked along Station Road and up to the common, along a path in front of some cottages until we reached the village hall. In Station Road there were two places of interest, one for everyone and a special one just for me. The former was the Smithy where we could sometimes watch the blacksmith shoeing horses. He would heat the horseshoe in his furnace till it glowed red then, holding it in his long handled tongs, dip it in water, making it sizzle like chips in a pan of hot fat, before placing it gently on the horse's hoof. Amazing how such a large, powerful animal would stand so obligingly still while the blacksmith, holding the horse's bent leg up between his knees, nailed the shoe in place.

The second treat in Station Road was sometimes seeing my Dad. He worked for The Premier Cooling Company whose work site was situated at the end of the path after crossing the railway line. The large wooden doors to the entrance were nearly always open and if I waited either Dad or one of his mates would see me and tell him I was there. It was great to have a wave from my Dad in the middle of my school day.

Prior to this employment Dad worked as a doorman at the new cinema in Guildford called the Astor. A visit to this cinema in the 1950s meant having the door opened for you by a uniformed doorman and an usherette would show you to your seat by the light of her torch. Between films, when the house lights were on, she would patrol the auditorium with a waist level tray of ice creams secured by a sash round her neck.

There was an air of luxury to the new Astor cinema: plush carpet, impressive lighting and large draping curtains, which slowly drew back in folding pleats to reveal the screen. In return for having the advertising film posters displayed on the double fronted wooden building adjacent to our house, we were allowed free seats at the Astor. I know I developed a love of films and cinema from regular visits with my Mum or friends. I saved some of my favourite posters for a long time and now wish I still had them – I had no idea they would one day become as collectable and valuable as they have done. If I remember rightly the first film shown at the Astor was the beautiful story of 'Gi Gi' with Maurice Chevalier, Hermione Gingold and starring Leslie Caron as Gi Gi. We went to see the film with Mum, and Dad was on duty in his burgundy uniform with brass buttons, and as an extra treat, we went in the Astor Bar upstairs for something to eat before the film show.

Another Hollywood film that was later to have a lasting effect on me was Gone With The Wind. I have seen this film many times but the first time I saw it I was completely captured by the splendour and drama of this epic movie. A dramatic love story set against the backdrop of the American Civil War, the script of the film provides several famous quotes, none more so than the opening lines implying that life is no more than a dream remembered, a civilisation gone with the wind. An apt reminder that nothing remains the same forever.

During my last term at primary school there was an exciting event held in our school hall one evening. The cosmetic company Elizabeth

Arden were holding a meeting to demonstrate and advertise their products. I hadn't actually started wearing make-up yet but I was thinking about it and was thrilled when Mum agreed that I could go. Imagine my surprise when I was selected from a hall full of girls and ladies to be their model for a make-up demonstration. I even remember the name of the lipstick they used: it was English Rose. No doubt I looked older than I was and my height reinforced that illusion.

Tillingbourne Secondary School where I was destined to attend was having some new classrooms built. They were not ready for use when I was due to go there so my classmates and I had an extra year at junior school. My birthday fell just after the start of term in September so I was almost 13 when I started at secondary school. Being one of the eldest in the class didn't bother me at all but by now it was obvious that I was taller than the average schoolgirl my age and I wasn't too happy about that.

The school subjects at Tillingbourne were much more interesting, and included general science, I've never forgotten the fascination of using Bunsen burners and pipettes and doing experiments with iron filings to illustrate magnetic fields. The Headmaster, Mr Pink, took us for science and I did quite well in this subject, achieving my RSA School Certificate. During a lesson one day, I bent down to pick something up and my knees gave out a loud 'crack'; Mr Pink was within earshot and told me I would be a fixture by the time I was twenty-one! He was far from right.

Our curriculum included domestic science to learn about hygiene, ironing and cookery. I once got a house point for my fish cakes but I knew my future did not lie in the catering world. One cannot live on fishcakes alone.

My favourite and best subject was needlework. I possessed some creative skills because I had learnt to knit some years before and had moved on from designing and knitting dolls' outfits to knitting my own jumpers. Now I was learning to make clothes in fabric.

Choosing a style from the big pattern catalogues of Simplicity, Style or Vogue was almost as exciting as choosing the fabric. The pleasure of selecting colours and textures has always stayed with me, and even now I love the need for new curtains – it's a reason to spend ages looking at fabric samples. I made lots of my own clothes after I left school, especially as the shift dress style of the early sixties was very easy to make, but I also liked the challenge of something more tailored with a collar and lining. It was just as well that I did, as my GSE 'O' Level exam in dressmaking included having to set a sleeve into an armhole. I felt a great sense of pride and satisfaction when I achieved a pass and got my dressmaking 'O' level with a credit.

I certainly wasn't the only girl who made her own clothes at school and an end of term highlight was a fashion show where we all wore outfits that were our own creations. To our delight this event was featured in the local newspaper, complete with photographs. During my last year at school, the company who made the Style range of patterns visited the school with lots of their creations for us to put on a fashion show. Imagine, a class of fifteen year old girls being models. We were all given tips on grooming (removing leg and underarm hair). I remember being selected to wear a summer outfit with shorts because my legs were all right. Gosh, I thought they were just too long!

Fortunately, English Language was my second best subject. I liked learning about the use of words and took pleasure in writing essays or stories. I clearly remember coming out of my GSE 'O' Level English Language exam thinking, whether I pass or not, I really enjoyed that exercise. I am pleased to say that I did pass.

I was content to be in the top stream at school and do the best I could. Just as well I had no dreams of ever going to university to become something professional, though I gained my modest RSA School Certificate by passing five subjects altogether: English Language, Maths, Arithmetic, General Science and Needlecraft.

Education was now being geared to training for the big wide world and the prospect of earning our own living. I joined the Commerce class and Mrs Bothamley taught us to touch type on the heavy manual typewriters. In our needlework class those who were learning to type made covers for our keyboard. It went over our heads like an apron and tied round the back of the typewriter, covering the keys. With our hands completely hidden we learned the entire 'qwerty' keyboard. Our fingers blindly becoming so familiar with the location of the letters of the alphabet we were eventually able to type text with a continuous rhythm and speed. 'The quick brown fox jumps right over the lazy dog' and 'now is the time for all good men to come to the aid of the party' were our practice lines, the former using every letter of the alphabet. What a skill! I thought it was great and I really enjoyed it.

Alongside the typing Mrs Bothamley also taught Pitman's shorthand. I look back on this as one of the biggest challenges of my life. Firstly we learned the Pitman's Shorthand alphabet. Fine, this was quite easy, but then vowels, diphthongs and shortforms were added, lines were either thick or thin and placed above, on or through the line depending on the vowel. Every word in any language could be written in lines, circles, hooks or curves. Help! It was an overwhelming jumble of nonsense to me. I even considered the possibility of giving up as I thought it was beyond my comprehension until, one day, it all started to fall into place and make sense. Hooray! I had cracked it. This seemed an even more impressive skill to me and I soon enjoyed taking dictation and typing it back, practising, faster and faster. I was one of a small group who attended extra classes at Mrs Bothamley's house for dictation practice. What a lovely generous teacher she was to go that extra mile for her pupils, I for one certainly appreciated it. I wasn't the best in the class but I achieved my RSA certificate for dictation at a respectable speed of 80 words per minute.

When I was fourteen I had a Saturday job and worked in Freeman Hardy &Willis, a shoe shop in Guildford. Each shop assistant had a duplicate receipt book and every time we sold a pair of shoes we would write out a receipt for the customer. On my first day I had no idea how busy it was going to be but I seemed to be selling shoes like hot cakes. The shop was buzzing all day and I recall the Manager's amazement and almost disbelief, when I showed him my total sales for the day. We were paid commission on our sales, I don't recall how much I got but I know I did very well that day.

I'm not sure exactly why I changed my Saturday job but I later went to work for Marks & Spencer's, also in Guildford. At least I didn't have to keep bending down to put down and pick up pairs of shoes from the floor. Self-service style of retailing had not yet been introduced so there was much interaction between sales assistant and customer and I enjoyed this job much more, working in ladies' fashion, selling jumpers.

At that time the Odeon Cinema in Guildford often hosted musical celebrities. It was the early 1960s and rock, pop and skiffle groups were everywhere. One group who seemed to be growing in popularity and making a name for themselves was booked to perform at the Odeon. They were four young men, dressed in black suits and all sporting similar fringed hairstyles. One Saturday I saw them as they walked through Marks & Spencer's – they were John, Paul, George and Ringo. Yes, it was the Beatles!

One of the benefits of being younger than my brother and sister was that I was fortunate enough to be in the right age group to go on the first trip abroad to be organised by Tillingbourne School. During the Easter holiday we were to visit Belgium and stay in the coastal town of Ostend. It is hard to imagine now just how amazing the prospect of not only leaving home but of actually leaving the country was.

On the day of departure I found it hard to eat my breakfast and could not understand why. When Mum said it was nerves because I was excited, it was the first time I had experienced such feelings. It was a great trip with many good memories including visiting the Atomium in Brussels and the tulip gardens of Keukenhof. For me the trip provided another abiding memory. An eighteen-year old young man and his parents were staying in the same residence as us and they joined our party on our coach trips. I was not yet interested in boys and certainly not looking for a boyfriend and yet there seemed to be an attraction between myself and the young man whose name was Martin. We talked and walked a lot together and found a mutual affection for each other. On the last day of our holiday, which was a Saturday, we had to say goodbye. I was fourteen and it was just a holiday friendship and yet parting was mutually painful. It was a poignant separation as he held me close and kissed me for the first time. I believed I had fallen in love for the first time.

It was good to be safely back home from my first trip abroad but the following few Saturdays were really miserable for me as I remembered my friendship with Martin and our sad farewell. My Mum was very understanding, she never said I was silly, stupid or too young and this helped me get over it but, of course, the memory stayed with me. As I grew older I often reminded myself never to belittle or underestimate the strength of feelings of a fourteen year old.

The criterion for a place on a secretarial course at Guildford Technical College in the early sixties was five 'O' levels. I was applying for such a position and my maths teacher, Mr McCormack, vouched for me saying I should be able to achieve the necessary passes. In the event, I only got two 'O' Level passes but to my delight was still admitted to the course. So I became a secretarial college student under the tuition of Mrs Wellington. That winter of 1962/3 proved to be one of the coldest and longest on record, snow lay deep and long. I was proud to wear my college scarf and glad of its woollen warmth as I walked from Guildford bus station to the college every day. I remember seeing the remains of a snowman in a garden one day – it was the first of April.

As I already had typing skills I had the privilege of being the first student to use the only electric typewriter available to the class while everyone else had to bash away on manual machines. It was the only time I ever felt more advanced than my fellow students. However, this privilege was relatively short lived, as it was only fair that everyone should have a turn on the mains powered appliance.

There were times, fortunately not too often, when I was made acutely aware that I was the only student from a secondary modern school in Mrs Wellington's class. The majority of girls on the course were very friendly even though their backgrounds were more well to do than mine. Our timetable had to include a foreign language and all the other students had already been learning another language but Tillingbourne School had had no such facility. I chose Spanish and attended extra evening classes as well to try and keep up. It was a struggle, as was Commerce and Law, so I decided to put most of my energies into my shorthand and typing. Anyway, I hoped to work in an office and had no ambition to become a travel agent, entrepreneur or a lawyer.

A very good friend at the time lived near Shere and belonged to Shere Youth Club; every month they had a Friday evening coach outing to Richmond Ice Rink. How exciting, I could go to her house straight after college and join the skating trip. I dressed appropriately on the day and wore my jeans to college. Oh my god, I might as well have worn my birthday suit! Mrs Wellington was stopped in her tracks when she saw me; what was I thinking of? A secretarial student, wearing jeans! When I explained that I was going ice skating in the evening straight from college, she addressed the whole class telling us that we were there to study, we did not have a social life for the year that we were her students, and we were to be dressed appropriately. Fifty years on I think she would be turning in her grave to know what students look like today and that jeans are actually allowed to be worn in some offices. Why do some teachers have such amazing names? Mrs Wellington aka The Old Boot!

The Richmond skating trips continued and I was making more friends, getting to know some of the other youth club members. One memorable evening the Youth Club assistant leader seemed very attentive and helped me round the rink as I slipped and slid on the ice. Christopher Dean he was not but he could skate better than me. His actual name was Colin Woolmington and I guess I was somewhat impressed as he seemed quite nice and at least he was tall. As we all boarded the coach for the journey home, I wondered if he would sit next to me. Being in charge of the outing he had to make sure everyone was on board before getting on the coach himself. By the time he walked up the coach, one of his mates had occupied the seat next to me. I said nothing, not wishing to be too presumptuous. Colin said nothing either and took the spare seat at the back of the coach. Maybe I was wrong and he hadn't enjoyed the evening as much as I had. I certainly didn't feel quite so happy on the journey back. I need not have worried: before we said goodbye that evening Colin asked if I would like to go out with him. We arranged our first date there and then. Wow! Before I knew it, I was courting.

The last term at college included preparation for interviews, hopefully leading to future employment. Mrs Wellington had many contacts in London who were very willing to employ girls who had been on her secretarial course, knowing they were 'of a very good calibre'. A group of us were sent to the head office of Courtaulds in London. There was only one vacancy so for all except one of us it was an exercise to gain interview experience. I wasn't too excited about the company – the only thing that appealed to me was the fact that they dealt with fabric and had bolts of material displayed in their reception, so I wasn't too disappointed not to get the job.

I decided to try and find a job myself and independently contacted an employment agency in London. Would this girl from a secondary modern school pass muster? Yes, I promptly secured a job with a firm of consulting engineers called R W Gregory & Partners. Their offices were on the first floor of Redland House in Kingsway, London WC2.

Before I started work, Mum and I had a trip to London. I was pleased to show Mum exactly where I would be going every day and it was good to have a dummy run of the journey. It was a very exciting time in my life but I understood my parents' concern for their seventeen-year old daughter, soon to become a commuter.

---o0o---

CHAPTER VI

Teen years and beyond

Arriving at Waterloo about 8.30am every day I would walk over Waterloo Bridge, across the Strand, round Aldwych and up Kingsway to where I worked. The first floor office was accessed via a lift with clanging, metal concertina doors. I shared the office with three other girls and we all got on very well. All the engineers were very nice and I enjoyed my job. Some of the typing was very challenging as this was long before the introduction of computers where there would no doubt have been a template to just fill in. Documents called 'distribution boards' which related to electrical installations required calculations to work out the width of each column to ensure all the characters and numbers fitted across the page and every mistake had to be erased and retyped correctly. Photocopiers were not yet available either, a fact that is making me feel very old, so 'masters' were typed on waxed stencils that were then fitted onto a Gestetner Duplicator to roll off the required number of copies. If an error occurred while typing a stencil the waxed top layer was held away from the backing sheet and red correcting fluid was painted over the error. When the fluid had dried the stencil was realigned in the typewriter and the correction made. As I type this and remember the procedure, I'm sure I can actually smell the correction fluid.

Only people educated in the pre-computer age can appreciate the revolutionary changes it has made to so many aspects of our lives and work.

One day, one of my colleagues who sat opposite me with her back to a tall window with long curtains, decided her stencil was beyond correction; she ripped it from her typewriter and threw it in the bin by her desk. Smoking was not banned in the workplace, or anywhere else, at that time and she obviously thought this seemed like a good time for a fag. She lit up her cigarette and tossed the match into the bin. Whoosh! The wax stencil burst into flames, which then leapt up the curtains. The whole event caused quite a stir in the office but fortunately we managed to beat the fire out before any real serious damage occurred. How times have changed: there wasn't even a smoke detector to set off an alarm. At least that meant we didn't disturb the whole building and we could keep our misadventure to ourselves.

One day when my colleagues were all ready to go home at the end of our working day they encouraged me to join them. I was reluctant because I had some work to finish for one of the engineers. However, I did join them and left the office but didn't feel comfortable about it. The next morning I was reprimanded not only for not finishing the work but more importantly for not telling the guy I was leaving the office without finishing it. Any pleasure of leaving work early with my colleagues was completely banished by my guilt. This was not an earth-shattering event by any means but I certainly learned to listen to and act by my own conscience in the future. Peace of mind is so valuable and good communication is vital.

The company employed a lady to do the filing; she was very thin and appeared quite old to me but was probably only in her late forties or early fifties. She would pop in from time to time to collect our file copies and, of course, have a chat. She would tell us of her man friend who used to visit her for sex. She seemed quite matter of fact about it and maybe she was just trying to impress us girls and prove that she wasn't past it.

Twice a day the clanging of the metal lift would be followed by the rattling of the tea trolley as the company tea lady wheeled her trolley into the office, offering much appreciated refreshments. Despite the fact that cream doughnuts were often on the menu and we often lunched out, I remained as tall and slim as ever. What a pity I never saw it as an asset, but never mind, it was great to be young, employed and have friends. The tea lady was always welcome as her arrival heralded a break for tea and a catch-up with the latest goings on in our lives. It was the tea lady who hinted to me one day that one of the young engineers was going to ask me out. How exciting! I had noticed him, he was quite good looking, had a good job, obviously, and had his own car! Oh my, I could have hit the jackpot here! Having a boyfriend who owned a car had not even entered my imagination: none of my friends had their own car so to have a boyfriend with a car was quite something in 1964. However, I was going out with Colin so I had a slight dilemma. I definitely would not two-time and date both of them.

The journey from Shere to my house in Shalford was about seven miles and Colin would often come over to see me after work as well as weekends. More than once we would overdo our goodbye and Colin would miss his last train and have to walk home – he must have been in love. The idea of calling a taxi never entered our heads as taxis were for rich people. Colin had a mate who lived near him and who also visited his girlfriend in my area and very occasionally he would see Colin walking home and give him a lift. One lovely summer evening as Colin and I were out walking in the village I told him about the chap at work and that I was considering going out with him. By the end of the evening my dilemma was solved. Having walked along the edge of the village green and stopped at a seat, we sat in the cooling evening air. Colin proposed to me and I said, "Yes".

I look back on those days with the fondest of memories. It was wonderful getting to know each other. We would often spend hours walking along the river or in the delightful local wooded hillside called the Chantries. We were lucky enough to have all this lovely countryside on our doorstep.

Many a summer Sunday afternoon we would hire a rowing boat and row along the river Wey from Guildford towards Godalming. When the weather was really good we would make an early start and catch a train to Portsmouth Harbour, hop onto the ferry, sail across the Solent and spend a day on the Isle of Wight. My work colleagues who mostly lived in London or Essex could hardly believe it when I told them where I had been on the weekend. I think we were so lucky to enjoy a proper courtship with the freedom to indulge in such outings together before the commitment and responsibilities of marriage.

Our monthly skating trips continued with the youth club. I don't think my skating improved much but it was always a great evening out. However, Friday night became the highlight of our week. One of Colin's mates had a Morris Eight car called Daisy, a genuine 1930s vintage model, sometimes referred to as a matchbox on wheels. It was certainly a cute model and with his girlfriend the four of us would pile in and set off for a pub called The Wooden Bridge in Guildford. Friday night was Rhythm and Blues night and who should be providing the live music? None other than Mick Jagger and the Rolling Stones, and sharing the bill was Long John Baldry. I still get a thrill to think how close I was to them while bopping with the crowd. The Beatles were good but to me The Rolling Stones will always be better. I loved the earthy sound of their music and adored Mick Jagger when he strutted his stuff – and he was tall and lean!

How well I remember one fateful Friday evening when a wheel fell off Daisy on the way home from The Wooden Bridge. I can't remember any technical details or how the others got home but I remember Colin walking me back to my house. It was very dark and very late and we were the only people in the road. As my home came into sight we could see the front bedroom window was open wide. "Where the devil have you been and hurry up and come in." Mum was obviously very worried – it wasn't like her to shout down the road. It was hilarious to us trying to explain that a wheel had fallen off the car and by the time we reached my door our humour had diffused my Mum's concern and she was also seeing the funny side of it. No doubt the relief that we were safe also had something to do with it.

Working in London and being a teenage bride in the 'swinging sixties' seemed quite sensational; I admit it was an exciting time. I loved the buzz of London then and I still do. A week or so before I left my job to get married the office secretary took me to John Lewis in Regent Street where I had the pleasure of choosing a wedding present from the company. We returned to our office by taxi with a beautiful, long, teak coffee table. I was thrilled; it was the first piece of furniture Colin and I owned and it was up-to-the-minute style for our new home.

The day I left my job in London the coffee table came home with me. The other girls had organised for a taxi from Kingsway to Waterloo and one of them came with me as a necessary escort. The taxi wasn't all that they had organised: my coat had been stuffed with confetti and I left a trail of it in my wake. I remember it littering the platform at Waterloo as the table and I were put on the train. I don't remember how I got home from Shalford station.

Our main concern while we had been engaged was where we were going to live. I came home from work one day to discover that Mum had been talking to the people who lived opposite us. Some friends of theirs had just moved into a three-storey house at number 15 Marshall Road, Godalming and were looking for tenants to occupy the flat on the top floor. We viewed the flat and the rest is history as they say. Colin had been living in lodgings in Shere so he moved into our flat straight away as we could not afford two lots of rent. I did not move in with him, 1964 was a time when respectability and a girl's reputation went hand in hand; it was definitely not the done thing.

Our wedding took place on Saturday 19 December 1964 at St Mary's church in Shalford. On the morning of that day I kept my hairdresser's appointment in Guildford and had a wander through Marks & Spencer's beforehand. One of the staff who I had known from when I worked there, asked what I was doing – wasn't I getting married that day? "Yes, I am," I said. I couldn't see a problem – I knew I'd be back in time to get ready.

It was a lovely wedding on a bright December day. As tradition dictated I had something old, something new, something borrowed and something blue. It's interesting how I remember some of the guests huddling in their coats against the cold when we came out of the church and yet I didn't feel at all cold in my white wedding dress. I also remember asking Colin to stop as we walked down the church path before we got into our hire car to go to the reception. I wanted to savour the moment, look around us and particularly remember that part of our day.

Our wedding was planned in six weeks and took place less than a week before Christmas Day. The guys at work were not alone in thinking that it was a 'shotgun wedding': my father-in-law was also suspicious of my condition. I confess to enjoying the intrigue until time proved them wrong; I was not pregnant. We did not have the time (or the money) to plan a honeymoon so we decided to spend our first night in London and so we stayed at the Strand Palace Hotel. A hotel we were to stay in again on our Ruby anniversary forty years later.

Colin and I had decided it would be sensible for me to work locally after our marriage. I was, indeed, enjoying the routine of life running to our own timetable. Not having to catch a train to and from work every day played a huge part in this freedom. It was also obviously much more economical but it did take a while for me to get used to, and appreciate the benefits of working locally and walking to work. Whenever I had a day off I would head to the station, catch a train to London and visit my old work colleagues. I had the best of both worlds. For Colin, it also meant not having to make the frequent journey over to see me. It was super to be together every evening and be able to say goodnight instead of goodbye.

Our new home was so conveniently situated we were within easy walking distance of all amenities including the cinema that then existed in Godalming. When Gone With The Wind was showing it was a 'must see' film. I had seen the film many times but Colin had not and it obviously didn't have the same effect on him. While I still wallowed in the story when we got home, expecting him to sweep me up in his arms, carry me into the bedroom and kick the door shut (just like Rhett Butler did with Scarlet O'Hara), Colin decided to watch Match of the Day on the television!

One Monday morning in January 1965, a few weeks after my wedding, I started work at Bookwise and South Country Libraries. The company was within walking distance of our flat and meant walking into Godalming and then down Catteshall Lane. To me at that time, it seemed a long, boring walk, no hustle and bustle of busy commuters off to their location in the City. I could not believe I even saw cows in a field by the river, had I really left London for this? This small town High Street was no comparison for Oxford Street or the Strand in my lunch hour!

Yes, it was a culture shock at first and I really missed working in London. I was still in touch with the girls in the office and the four of us had got on really well together. They missed me too and had a word with the Company Secretary. As a result, I was offered my old job back. I could work shorter hours and, in return, forfeit the end of year pay rise. It was an exciting prospect. I turned it over and over in my mind as I walked to work each morning, I had to give them an answer as quickly as possible. I considered talking to my

Mum about it but my circumstances had changed. I was a married woman now: I had to make my own decisions. I weighed up all the pros and cons and soon realised that coping with shopping, cleaning and housework whilst working full time was a pretty hefty schedule without adding two hours travelling every day. And that would be on a good day without any train delays or cancellations. Decision made, I grudgingly stuck with my local job and continued walking to work.

Every cloud has a silver lining, though. I shared an office with another shorthand typist called Pat and fortunately we hit it off together from the word go. The first time I saw her I thought she was younger than me; with her short blonde hair and pretty face she looked as fresh and lovely as Doris Day. Being quite chuffed with my new status I proudly told her I had been married for six weeks. She promptly replied that she had been married six years! Ye gods, I was a teenage bride, just how old was this girl? It transpired that she was engaged on her seventeenth birthday and married on her eighteenth. We became firm friends and soon suggested going out as a foursome with our husbands. Thanks to Pat, I grew to like working in Godalming, and it obviously had the benefit of a less stressful lifestyle with more free time to socialise with our new friends, Pat and Pete.

Our friendship was growing stronger but within a year, I chose to change my employment and went to work for a nearby company called RFD. This company manufactured ground-to-air missile training simulators, life rafts and escape chutes for aircraft. Many a time I have noted with great interest the RFD logo seen on my travels in later life. I was the secretary to the Assistant Sales Director and within weeks we were in his car heading for the annual Boat Show at Earls Court in London. It was my first experience of facing the general public, the majority of whom had a keen interest in boats. This job was certainly more interesting, with slightly shorter hours for more money but I still found Catteshall Lane very uninteresting.

After nearly two wonderful years of living in our flat, my parents decided they would like to have a more interesting role in their retirement. They became live-in handyman and companion to a lady who was the great-granddaughter of Thomas Cook (of travel fame) and lived in a lovely large house in Wonersh. How wonderful: going to visit them would mean an opportunity to revisit my childhood village. We thus moved into my parents' bungalow in Godalming, which we agreed to rent for the same rental we were paying for our flat. Of course, it was great to have our own front gate, front door and garden but somehow, for me, it was tinged with a slight sadness. I remember thinking that our romantic days of being a young flat-dwelling couple were over forever.

Nevertheless, it was a good move. We had more freedom to invite friends round and were even allowed to decorate to our own taste. Our first target was the lounge, a project Colin launched himself into with amazing enthusiasm. I agreed we should rub down the woodwork before painting and then paper the walls. Well, some of the woodwork was taken back to the bare wood and hairline cracks in the wall opened up, under Colin's attention, like mini grand canyons! I'll never be sure that this was really necessary but when filled the cracks were smoothly flush with the walls and the finish on the gloss painted woodwork was second to none.

Sharing our enthusiasm for our decorating project, dear Pat and Pete offered their assistance. Whether we were working fast to impress is doubtful but when they called round we had little left to do, apart from clearing up, but admire our freshly painted woodwork, especially the bay window sill. No matter, coffee and a chat is always a welcome excuse for a break. Pat had come prepared and promptly donned her 'marigolds' (rubber gloves), pushed up her sleeves and strolled over to the window. Planting her hands firmly on the still wet painted windowsill, she gazed out and announced, "Right, where do we start?"

While we were renting the flat we had acquired our first set of wheels, albeit only two of them. Yippee, we were mobile! We became proud owners of a Honda 50, complete with matching 'his' and 'hers' white, peaked crash helmets. At last we could enjoy the freedom of the open road but preferably in fine weather. We had a trip to the coast costing us 2/6d (25p) in petrol and I had to walk up Bury Hill because the two-stroke engine was not powerful enough to carry us both up the steep road over the South Downs. What an adventure that day was.

While we were renting my parents' bungalow Colin's Dad presented us with the opportunity of acquiring our first car. He had a black Ford Prefect on offer for the handsome sum of fifty pounds. This was more than half Colin's monthly salary but we decided to go ahead and purchase it. Colin travelled on a one-way train ticket to his parents in Essex and returned home at the wheel of his very own car.

What excitement, where should we go? We very soon made plans to go west for a camping holiday. With our luggage on board and a tent kindly loaned to us by our friends and neighbours, the young couple who lived next door, we were ready to hit the road. Unfortunately our Ford Prefect was not as ready as we were: it refused to move. Luckily our friendly neighbours were on hand to give us a send-off so they gave us a push as well. Did it bode well to set off for Wales, I asked myself, with our neighbours pushing and running alongside us as we chugged down the road?

We journeyed as far as Shepton Mallet in Somerset where we pitched up for an overnight stop. Our accommodation was a ridge tent, which we had not bothered to investigate too closely. No doubt our neighbours were not aware or had completely forgotten, that one of the main tent poles was broken. Never mind, we just had a tent with a much higher roof at one end!

Our initial start should have warned us of problems ahead. The next morning, after breakfast, we were packed and ready to go.

Again the Prefect had other ideas and again refused to start. This was the 1960s, an era when young couples did not openly go away together unless they were married. Although we were feeling rather conspicuous, a young couple, obviously not having the wherewithal to buy a decent tent, not to mention a decent car, it was also quite amusing. I'm sure we drew a few disapproving tuts from behind closed tent flaps but we had nothing to be embarrassed about other than a dysfunctional car.

Thank goodness, it was also an era when men tinkered with their cars as part of proving their masculine ability to fix things. So it was that several mature, male campers gathered round our stricken vehicle like bees round a honey pot. The bonnet was up, their heads were down, it was remedy by committee. Personally I have no idea what they did but they fixed it for us. Profusely expressing our gratitude and to our great relief, we finally drove off on the next leg of our adventure.

The second Christmas after we got married, we were guests of Pat and Pete for the festive season. Staying with friends for Christmas was lovely and we had a super time together. Fortunately, we all had understanding parents who accepted this arrangement.

When Pat's sister, her Mum and her family had a holiday on the Isle of Wight, we popped over on the ferry from Portsmouth to spend a day with them. It was a lovely, sunny day out with plenty of time spent on the beach. "Watch out, Colin's getting broody," yelled Pat as Colin enjoyed playing with her young niece. "I hope not," I retorted. "I'm not ready yet!"

We had many more trips to the Isle of Wight with Pat and Pete. Having found a cosy B&B in Shanklin, run by a Miss Parfitt who originally came from Guildford, we prolonged our days out to weekends away. We were staying there on the memorable date in July 1969 when Apollo 11 landed on the moon and Neil Armstrong was the first man to walk on the moon. It seemed incredible to be able to actually watch this historic event on television.

How apt that our first ever flight destination was to be with Pat and Pete. Foreign holidays were still relatively new on the scene but that didn't stop us speculating about the possibility of having a holiday abroad together. It seems very cautious now but the destination we decided on was the Channel Island of Jersey. We booked a two-week, full board, holiday in The Merton Hotel in St Helier. I now marvel at the fact we could afford it, whilst we were saving for a house. Thank goodness we did – it was a glorious holiday, full of sun, sand and sea and lovely memories.

We flew from Shoreham Airport in West Sussex, excitedly (for me) and nervously (for Colin) boarding the little plane for the short 140 mile flight. All went smoothly until, nearing the end of our journey when we experienced turbulence! It certainly wasn't the smoothest of landings, not rough enough to spoil our holiday but rough enough to dampen my excitement at the prospect of flying home. I remember feeling quite edgy on our last day. I like to think it didn't show and that our friends didn't realise why I wanted to walk away from them and spend time on our own rather than risk falling out with them.

I really believe the sun shone every day for two whole weeks of our holiday. We spent many days on the beach soaking up the sun and many evenings in the bars soaking up every kind of cocktail imaginable. After a game of beach football one day Colin's sunburnt feet swelled so painfully he couldn't get his shoes on for a couple of days. I remember visiting a strawberry farm and sitting on a wall in the sun, experiencing the pleasure of eating the beautiful, ripe fresh fruits whilst enjoying the company of our best friends.

We continued our outings with Pat and Pete in their car as our new wheels were hardly reliable enough to risk taking passengers out with us. On one occasion even the driver's side window, which was operated by a handle to wind it up or down, decided to malfunction.

The window just dropped down inside the doorframe and refused to reappear no matter how much the winder handle was turned. Even so, these were mortgage-free carefree days. I still believe I was born and grew up at the best time ever. The war had ended and despite the initial austerity before too long society seemed to be enjoying greater freedom and prosperity than it had for years.

Another employment change opportunity arose when my Mum showed me an advertisement she had spotted in the local newspaper for an "attractive secretary". In the light of modern social acceptance and political correctness, the thought of that now makes me cringe. The company was in the High Street, a location that had much more appeal to me. I applied for and got the post and for the next twenty-two and a half years worked for the business agents Ronald A Rawlings Ltd.

We may not have been working together any more but that certainly didn't have a detrimental effect on my friendship with Pat. In fact, quite the reverse: our relationship deepened and the four of us were frequently socialising. Consequently, we were introduced to one of their favourite haunts, a Berni Inn in Wokingham called the Old Rose. Berni Inns were a very popular chain of restaurants in the sixties. We were always very grateful that our friends were kind enough to take us in their car whenever we went out together. We actually owned very little at the time; our rented accommodation was furnished so we hadn't had the necessity to acquire our own material trappings of home life, other than clothes. In contrast, our new friends had had six years in which to establish themselves in their own home with their own furniture and a car; excellent role models for us to aspire to. We enjoyed having other friends to visit us but I think we were so lucky to have met Pat and Pete so early in our married life. They were a super, genuine, sociable couple, and they smoothed the way for us to integrate into our new abode and lifestyle. Quite often we would be joined by more of their friends, which was wonderful and meant we had a really good social circle.

One evening at the Old Rose we were to be introduced to Pat and Pete's friends Rita and Bob. It was always good to dress well when going out for a meal and on this occasion we made a bit of an effort, it was the 1960s and not over-the-top for Colin to wear a suit – even the suit he got married in.

We drank schooners of sherry, and dined on the ubiquitous menu of the time: prawn cocktail, steak and chips, and Black Forest gateau. The six of us got on really well and had a brilliant evening together. Before leaving the Old Rose, Pat and Pete invited us all round for coffee at their place. What a great idea, back to theirs to round off our lovely evening.

It was no surprise that Colin and Pete wanted to stop for a convenience break on the way home. We weren't far from home but they definitely could not wait for a pee, nor apparently could Bob who was also grateful for the stop. So it was that we came to be parked on a stretch of road, which had just crossed the river and was flanked on either side by open meadowland. It was not far short of midnight and from a clear, star twinkling sky, a full moon illuminated the scene.

Three smartly dressed young men walked several yards ahead where there was a short stretch of railings along the edge of the road. Pete held the railings, stepped cautiously over them and moved carefully along to the privacy of some small trees. Colin threw caution to the wind, vaulted over the railings, easily clearing them but then disappearing from sight amidst a confusion of splashing and swearing! In answer to Pete's request as to where Colin was, an almost frantic Colin shouted, "Down here in two foot of bloody water!" Did he swear or did he say muddy water? It really didn't make any difference: my husband was sitting upright in a ditch, wearing his best suit, in the moonlight.

We were all young and carefree and after our great evening of wining and dining we naturally found this happening hilariously entertaining. Even Colin's sense of adventure was only slightly tempered by his damp, cold discomfort. Our hysterical laughter echoed around the darkness. The sight of Colin, who had managed to clamber out of the ditch, walking awkwardly towards us only served to enhance our entertainment; we were all completely helpless with laughter.

Our resourceful friends had the foresight to carry a rug in their car so eventually, suitably wrapped, Colin was allowed back into their vehicle and we travelled on to our flat. Yes, we were going to Pat and Pete's for coffee but not with Colin dressed like that. When he stripped off for a quick dip in the bath, the full extent of his 'adventure' was revealed. The colour of his suit disguised much of the mud but the same could not be said for his underwear, what a mess. Guess who had the job of taking his suit to the cleaners?

Suitably clean and clad in another suit (the one time in his life Colin owned two suits), we all resumed our journey for coffee at Pat and Pete's place. It wasn't our last outing with Rita and Bob but I can't help wondering what kind of first impression we had made on them.

---oOo---

CHAPTER VII

Home owners

After several years of careful money management and diligent saving, Colin and I were able to consider buying our own home, and in 1968 we purchased a three bedroom semi-detached house high on a hill overlooking Godalming. We had a very long terraced garden and the most wonderful distant views. Since getting married we had lived in furnished accommodation so we had very little stuff to move. Our friend Pete generously agreed to move us so all our personal possessions including our coffee table were loaded onto his company lorry and delivered to our new address.

Stripped of all its furnishings our new home did not seem as welcoming as when we had viewed and chosen it. No matter, it was ours and we soon got settled in with two deck chairs in the lounge plus our coffee table, a new bed and a kitchen table and chairs purchased from the previous residents. Having made this commitment we were happily settled and looked forward to furnishing our new home and maybe then starting a family.

We also decided a more reliable car was necessary and purchased a second-hand blue Austin Cambridge with a white flash. What a contrast to our little Prefect; it seemed huge and quite luxurious. Before having official lessons Colin often took me out driving so I could get familiar with this exciting mode of transport. When I was instructed to reverse round a left hand corner during my driving test the car started to run backwards because I had not realised I was reversing down a hill. Luckily I had the presence of mind to ask if I could repeat the exercise and promptly did so perfectly. Ever since I always tell myself that making a mistake does not mean failing – it's the way you handle the mistake that counts. I passed my driving test at the first attempt.

Getting pregnant didn't happen as quickly as I imagined but eventually our family was on the way. How exciting: we were due to have a Christmas baby, the expected date of arrival being 23 December 1970. There was snowfall that December and I remember being heavily pregnant and very carefully picking my way through the icy, sludgy snow as I made my way home along our road.

Christmas Day and Boxing Day both came and went, New Year's Day came and went and I was still not a mother. At my next doctor's appointment I was told that if nothing had happened by the following Saturday I would be taken in and induced. A week later in the very early hours of the Saturday morning my baby let me know she was ready to start her journey into the world – could she have heard what had been said?

She may have been over two weeks late but our daughter Katherine Heather was certainly worth the wait. The prettiest and best behaved baby in the whole hospital and that is true. As was the norm at the time I had ten days in hospital following the birth and made the most of it. I still marvel at and wonder about the wisdom of mums taking their newborn babe home within hours of giving birth.

Now working in my third local job in Godalming it proved to be the best of all so far. Maternity leave was not a recognised legal right in 1971; in fact it was still not unknown for women to be sacked from their job just for being pregnant. Several weeks after our daughter was born it was arranged that I could still work for the company. I was supplied with an electric typewriter to work with from home and also worked Saturday mornings in the office. This brilliant agreement gave me some financial independence and meant I kept in touch with office life while also giving Colin some Daddy time with his daughter. This arrangement lasted for five pre-school years, after which I then went back to the office on a part-time basis and had school holidays off. The baby clinic, the playgroup and the junior school were all within walking distance of home, so life was not only very good, it was convenient too. How fortunate was that?

Like any family, holidays were very important to us. We bought a caravan and towed it around Britain at every opportunity. The Gower Peninsular in Wales, the Lake District and the Cotswolds were our favourite haunts. Another much frequented destination nearer home was our old stomping ground, the Isle of Wight. I absolutely adored the simple freedom of caravan living. It was like playing house.

In the late seventies, the then Prime Minister Harold Wilson visited the Isles of Scilly just off the coast of Cornwall, really putting them in the news. Colin suggested we should also visit the 'fortunate isles' as they were also called and so we seized the opportunity when our daughter went to camp with the Brownies. We took a train to Penzance, took the ferry to the main island of St Mary's, then a tractor ride to the campsite. It was an amazing adventure and despite enduring a force eight gale one night, the charm of the islands had completely captured us. We still return every year, occasionally even twice a year, almost forty years on.

Many years later Colin planned a November long weekend away. We were to stay in a castle in Cornwall – how exciting was that? We drove through the night, arriving at the Cornish coast to see the sunrise behind St Michael's Mount. It was beautiful. It was too early to book in to our accommodation so Colin suggested having a coffee at Penzance heliport. It was also too early for the café to be open but I got chatting to the lady who was getting everything ready to open up for the day. We practically told each other our life stories and I told her how excited I was to be staying in a castle in Cornwall. Time just flew by while we were chatting and when she was ready to serve coffee I suddenly realised Colin wasn't there. I looked around and saw him walking past the window. Was something wrong? Why was he going in the wrong direction?

A uniformed member of staff approached; I braced myself for the worst. I was handed two cards. What was going on? I couldn't understand the situation and where was Colin? The man in the uniform explained that I was holding boarding cards for the helicopter flight to the Scillies. It's hard to believe what an emotional surprise that was for me, like one of those moments when someone discovers their best friend is really their sister. At this point Colin returned with the rest of our luggage and confirmed we were indeed flying to St Mary's. Consumed with several emotions simultaneously I didn't know whether to laugh or cry so I started to shake and tremble. The man in the uniform said I had no need to worry, he would be coming with us; he was the pilot.

A birthday surprise one year started with another journey westward. Taking a break near Weymouth confirmed that we were not heading for Penzance this time. Hints were dropped about heights and views – was I really going to do a parachute jump? It transpired that we were actually going to catch the ferry to Guernsey. Very exciting but once again we were too early to book into our accommodation. Our luggage went into storage on the quay and we had a lovely day exploring St Peter Port, Guernsey. When we returned to the quay for our luggage Colin said he wanted to check something in the office. "Why?" Apparently he was picking up tickets for another boat trip! We weren't staying on Guernsey at all. We actually spent four heavenly days on the tiny island of Sark and visited the even smaller gem of an island called Herm. The sun shone every day as we wandered and cycled around our private paradise. It was beautiful and unforgettable.

Cycling had always been an important part of my life and when my old second-hand bike was replaced I became the delighted owner of a black and gold Raleigh Richmond Lady lightweight ladies touring bicycle. Although I was a very enthusiastic cyclist with many miles under my belt I wasn't that good at cycling uphill. A major problem was the fact that we lived at the top of a hill, good for the outward journey but not so good coming home. As an alternative to the hill I could take a shortcut involving ninety-two steps – even more reason for having a lightweight machine. I wonder how many times I have carried my bike up those steps over the years.

When our daughter was about six or seven years old sleepovers replaced babysitting with her friend Jane who lived nearby. They were much more fun for the girls and much better for the parents. One such morning I woke very early and looked out to soak up the wonderful view from our bedroom window in the early morning light. Colin had gone downstairs to make a cup of tea and he called up to me, "How about an early bike ride?" Wow, an opportunity not to be missed. I guessed it was about 8.00am and I was out of my jimjams, washed and ready and on my bike in a flash.

Being high summer it was pleasantly warm despite the early hour. The roads were virtually deserted but a few miles into our ride we saw a milkman doing his doorstep delivery. Those were the days when milk appeared like magic on our doorstep every morning. When we cycled past a village church, Colin drew my attention to the steeple with a church clock; he also rode alongside me with his wristwatch facing me. Did I notice the time? No, I had given up wearing a watch years before and was just enjoying my ride and the novelty of riding early in the morning. We rode at least twenty miles and passing an open baker's shop on the way home we decided a treat was deserved so bought some naughty buns for a breakfast feast when we got back. It was still too early to fetch our daughter when we got home. I wonder if we took advantage of being alone? Mmm funny how I don't remember that but I certainly remember the bike ride and the buns!

By the way, Colin had changed all our clocks (except his watch) and we had actually left home on our bikes at 6.00am!

That was by no means the only time that bicycles played a pivotal part in my life. My long held desire for a Caribbean holiday was frustrated by Colin's lack of enthusiasm for the same. Even on our twenty-fifth wedding anniversary I failed to win him over so years later when my fiftieth birthday loomed and he was planning a surprise holiday what else could it be but a sunshine trip to the Caribbean?

How wrong can you be? After weeks of teasing and excited anticipation I could hardly contain myself when Colin told me to look under my placemat at dinner one evening. Was it a trick? Was it a joke? It was certainly not tickets to the Caribbean. It was membership of the Youth Hostel Association! I was shocked and at a loss to understand until Colin explained we were going on a cycling youth hostelling holiday to the Isle of Wight. I was speechless and it took me all of two minutes before I could speak. Having processed my disappointment I felt energised and enthusiastic at the prospect of this surprise adventure.

It did in fact turn out to be a wonderful holiday. My first ever taste of hostelling and I was impressed; at least we had our own room and did not have to share a dormitory with strangers. We broke the ride to Portsmouth by staying a night at the Arundel hostel and then after the ferry trip, stayed at Sandown before riding right across the island to Totland Bay.

What a triumph. No doubt we would have had a lovely holiday in the Caribbean but I doubt we would have had the same feeling of achievement and I could still dream...

Unlike me Colin was sporty and very competitive. In fact he played so many sports I often said he would go out with the wrong bat one day. However, he won me over to join the local tennis club when he told me they had a sociable beginners section with chat and coffee time as well as tennis. I had no real experience of such clubs but by reputation believed they were all very cliquey. However, I joined the club and never looked back. Friendships forged over racquets and coffee have lasted a lifetime and the social spin offs were great.

When an opponent on the court one day was wearing a London to Brighton Bike Ride T-shirt I was on the case, full of questions and wanting to know more. The following year I was one of the twenty-seven thousand riders in the British Heart Foundation London to Brighton Bike Ride. I remember wondering if it was wise for me to be doing this challenge at my age of thirty-nine. That first ride was a very exciting personal challenge but the whole concept of raising money for a worthwhile cause whilst enjoying one of my best days ever was pretty addictive. So much so that I entered again the following year, the fact that I had travelled from London to the south coast entirely under my own pedal power felt like a truly amazing achievement.

I decided to make it a hat-trick and entered again for a third year. This time when I took my sponsor form round to my work colleagues some of them began showing great interest in the event. The result was that I organised a company team to enter the event the following year. Thereafter it became an annual event and I soon had all my contacts in place for hiring the vehicle and driver, arranging parking in Brighton and having a friend who stayed in all day so that anyone on the ride with a problem could ring her and then I would check with her from a phone box to see if there were any delays. The mobile phone, as we now know it, had yet to be invented.

Always on a Sunday in June, The London to Brighton Bike Ride invariably fell on Father's Day, which showed how committed everyone was to do the ride. Maybe there were some father and offspring riders amongst them. The first anniversary of my mother's death was on the same day as the bike ride in 1992 so I decided to give it a miss that year and spend the day with my Dad. However, Colin had a better idea: I did the ride and he brought Dad to Brighton in the car. It was brilliant to meet them both in the huge milling crowd on the seafront at the end of the ride and Dad, at the age of eighty nine, even had a little ride along the prom on my bike.

I have never been seriously athletic but this bike ride event really captured my imagination and I took it seriously. Preparation began about March or April every year with longer and longer rides at every opportunity. When I was working part-time I would often go out for the day with a packed lunch, enjoying the thrill of travelling thirty or forty miles as part of my training.

I thought I might call it a day after my twentieth ride. My sixtieth birthday and retirement was on the horizon and I felt it would be unfair to spend so much precious time out on my own when Colin and I stopped working. It was a hard decision because I still loved my annual day out to the seaside. To soften the blow I decided to ride one more time and this time I would not organize and enter as a team. The camaraderie had been wonderful every year but I thought it would be great to enjoy the event without having to think about booking and arranging payment for transport and parking and also not wondering how the others were doing and waiting for everyone to arrive in Brighton. If you were in the team you would probably laugh at that – I was usually the last one to arrive.

On the day of my final ride Colin drove me to Clapham Common with my bike and watched me disappear among thousands of pedals and helmets to join the hundreds of cyclists with whom I shared a start time. Dare I say I had the time of my life the day I rode my bike from London to Brighton on my own with twenty-six thousand, nine hundred and ninety-nine other cyclists. Always having a fellow rider to share stories with at every refreshment stop or hill walk, whether it was their first time or had they done the ride before, and if so how many times?

During the 1980s redundancy had become a familiar word in our vocabulary and rumours began to circulate about the future of The Gomshall Tannery. Colin had started his career in the grocery trade but had been working at the Tannery since before we met. We had both been very fortunate with our jobs and felt very secure with no big financial worries. We had more than two uncertain years of wondering whether the Tannery would close, though, our biggest worry being whatever would we do if it did.

One of the saddest days in my husband's life was Thursday 21 June 1988, the last day he was employed by The Gomshall Tannery. Now it was our turn to endure all the emotions and problems thrown up by redundancy. It was far more than just a job – after almost thirty years it was his way of life and work colleagues were a huge part of that life.

Despite my misgivings, purchasing a wholesale food distribution company in partnership with a couple of friends did solve our immediate employment issue. Reluctantly I left my lovely job after twenty-two and a half years with the company, justifying my sacrifice by telling myself it was worth it for us both to be working again.

In a nutshell, or maybe an eggshell, the business involved delivering mainly eggs and mushrooms to shops, take-a-ways, schools and nursing homes, etc. Put like that it sounds okay but this business had about two hundred and fifty customers, many of who had deliveries more than once a week. It was a big commitment and responsibility and sadly for me, a lifestyle I did not care for.

Regrettably this venture proved to be a bad move for me. I felt like I had been tipped out of the nest without a safety net. I was so far out of my comfort zone I began to dislike my life and was finding it difficult to cope. One of the worst moments I remember was when Colin and I were delivering to a take-away late one evening and we witnessed a fight in the high street of a local town. It was certainly not my idea of a way to earn a living and I was so glad my parents didn't know all that was involved in our business. I was definitely not dealing very well with our occupation and I saw my doctor for advice and promptly got an appointment with a counsellor. This proved to be very helpful, enabling me to get the situation in perspective and realise that it would not last forever. I was suffering the bitter taste of bereavement. No one had died but I was grieving for my old way of life.

There was no plan B: without the business Colin and I would both be unemployed but my faith in us finding further employment was much stronger than my faith in ever coming to terms with our current situation. The sale was not without its problems and hiccups but miraculously we managed to sell our business after about eighteen months. Yes, that left us both unemployed – what would we do now? It might sound like we made a reckless decision but after what we had been through we decided to go away in our caravan to the Lake District for a desperately needed break. After eighteen months without even a weekend off we felt we deserved it. It felt even better when Colin secured another job just before we went away – can you imagine the joy of that?

On a walk in the foothills near Wastwater Lake we came upon a little waterfall tumbling into a rock pool before flowing on into the lake. We were alone, the sun was shining, it was November, the beauty of our surroundings was uplifting and we had something to celebrate. My only regret is that Colin did not join me in skinny-dipping in the rock pool. He might have appreciated the view but I think he missed the most amazing experience of every aspect of freedom.

I started job hunting as soon as we returned and discovered to my bewilderment that computers were replacing typewriters. I was desperate to hone my skills and come up to date. I went to evening classes to learn about this new technology and I was even allowed back in the office of my old company so that I could get some practice. How generous was that? Before long I found a temporary full-time job in Godalming and when they asked me to stay on their permanent staff I jumped at it. It was an international firm of consulting engineers called Kennedy & Donkin, with lots of lovely employees and a social club.

One of the social club activities really appealed to me: it was ice-skating. I enjoyed it so much that another secretary and I decided to take lessons. The idea of gliding confidently on the sparkling white ice fired my imagination and I was eager to learn. My first lesson began with fearless enthusiasm and ended in the A and E department of the Royal Surrey Hospital. I had managed to fall over backwards and crack my head on the ice. As soon as I had healed I returned to the rink, joining the beginners' class and wearing a helmet for future lessons. I wanted to skate properly and, after all, it was how I had met Colin and I had paid for the whole term.

Wondering whether the age of fifty-two was a bit late to take up skating, a friend reassured me, saying I could still be a skater but maybe not a very good one. Of course I could, I didn't want to earn a living at it I just wanted to enjoy it. How glad was I that I pursued my interest and learned to skate properly. I learned that skates had an inside and an outside edge and by employing these edges correctly I became capable of doing cross-overs, chassis and turns, and to my delight, I could also perform these movements while skating backwards. What an achievement and the crowning glory for me was when I joined the cast in three consecutive Christmas pantomimes on ice at Guildford Spectrum sports centre.

This was more like it! I loved my job and the people I worked with. I really felt back on track and life was good again. I didn't know it at the time but the next few years were to hold some momentous events in my life and it was a great help and relief to be working for a supportive, compassionate company.

---o0o---

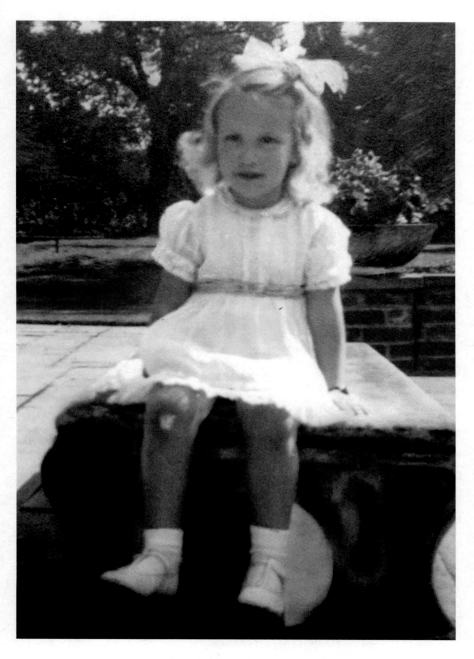

Me at age three. On the veranda at The Chase, Wonersh
where we lived in the servants' quarters

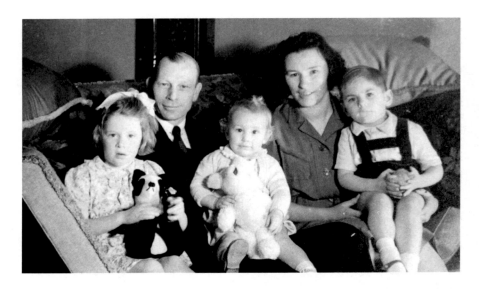

My sister Veronica (Vron to me), me sitting on Dad's lap and my brother Geoffrey (Geoff)
sitting on Mum's lap. Taken in the mid 1940s while we lived at The Chase, Wonersh, Surrey

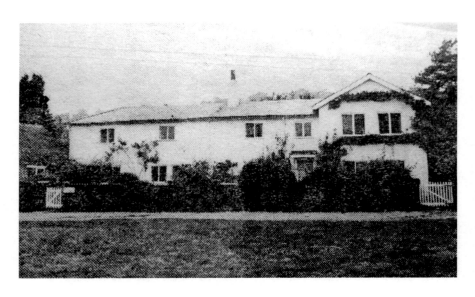

Meadow View, our lovely family home in the lovely Surrey
village of Wonersh where we lived for over ten years

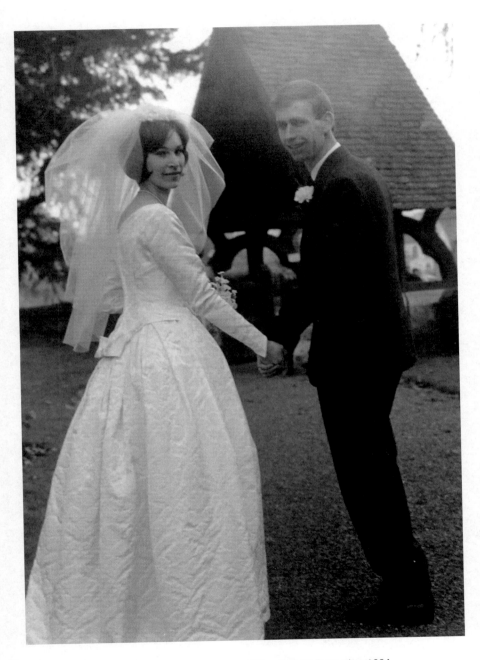

Our moment in time on our wedding day, 19 December 1964.
We married at St Mary the Virgin Church in Shalford, Surrey.

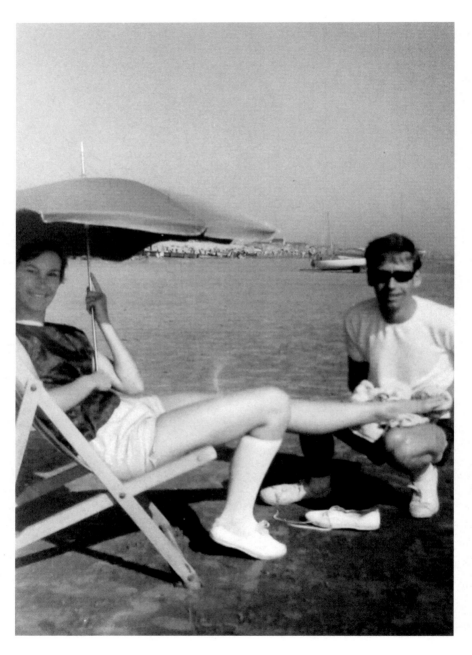

Carefree courting days in 1963. One of our many days out,
enjoying the sun, sand and beach on the Isle of Wight

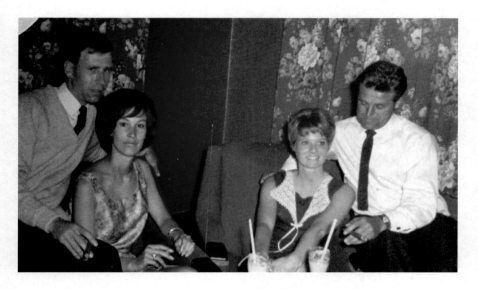

The first time we flew to our holiday destination. 1966 two beautiful fun filled weeks in Jersey with our wonderful friends Pat and Pete.

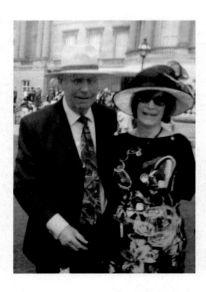

Colin and I at the Queen's Garden Party, Buckingham Palace on 1 June 2017. What an honour, thanks to the Kent Surrey and Sussex Air Ambulance for putting our names forward

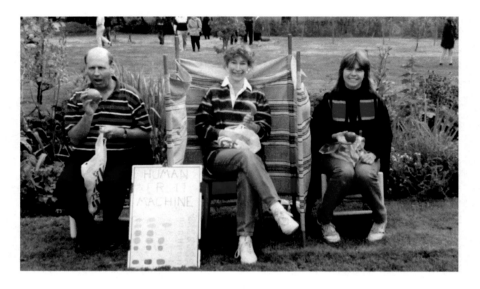

*I'm the banana in the middle. With Colin and our special friend Julie,
being a Human Fruit Machine at a Samaritans event in Guildford*

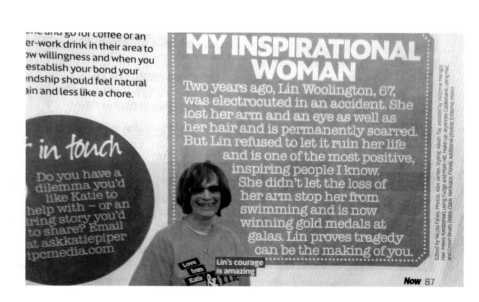

*A quote from Katie Piper, The Katie Piper Foundation.
This appeared in a copy of Now magazine in 2014*

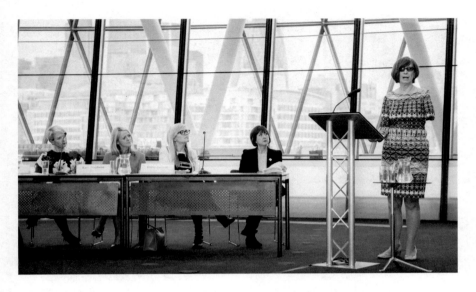

Telling my story in the Chamber of City Hall in London. An empowering event, I felt proud to represent The Katie Piper Foundation for International Women's Day

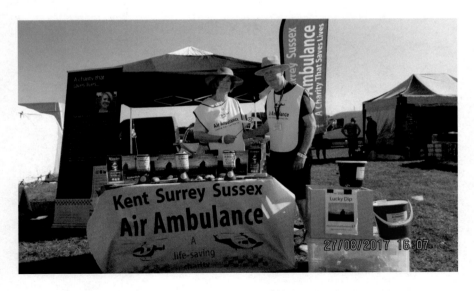

Colin and I running the Kent Surrey and Sussex Air Ambulance stall at the 2017 Wings and Wheels event in Dunsfold, Surrey. An event I always wanted to attend; it did not disappoint

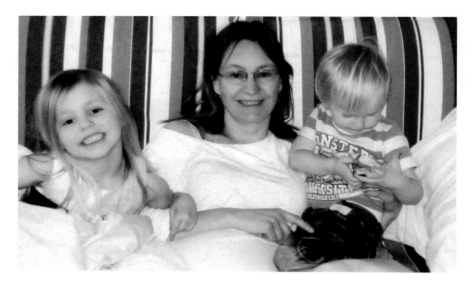

My beautiful daughter Katherine with her beautiful children Jennifer and Jack. Being a grandparent is one of the best experiences of my life

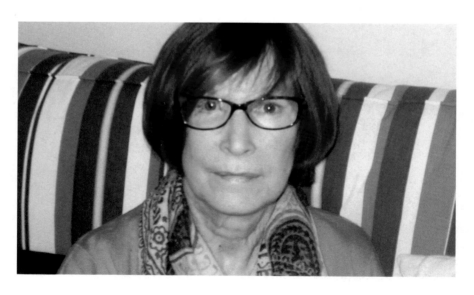

Me in 2017 after all my reconstructive operations. I think the experts did a pretty good job – I'm happy

CHAPTER VIII

Coping with grief

In 1991 my mother died. Mum had not fully recovered from her latest back operation several months earlier. She had become rather panicky and poor Dad was struggling to cope. Luckily we lived nearby and were able to frequently pop round at short notice to offer support and reassurance, even in the night when Dad sometimes rang in despair.

Following a successful Christmas coach holiday in Austria we booked up again to go in the summer. As our holiday date drew near we grew more and more anxious about leaving Mum and Dad for a week. We considered cancelling our trip but Mum agreed she would stay in a rest home while we were away, which would also give Dad the rest he so needed.

Everything was arranged and Mum duly went to the home the day before we were going away. While I waited for Colin to come home from work I decided to ring the home and see how Mum was settling in. I was totally unprepared for the sound of my tearful Mum asking me to get her out of there – she wasn't ready for an old people's home and would I come and fetch her. I tried to reassure her saying everything would be all right and it was only for one week. Ending the call I burst into tears of frustration and impotence

– what do I do now? Should we cancel the holiday? I had to dilute and share my emotions; I rang my Mum's doctor who had been in on the arrangement, surely she could help? Again I was totally unprepared for the response: "What do you expect me to do about it?" What was she saying? Was this her response to my dilemma? She's a doctor, surely she can help sort it out!

Colin arrived home equally unprepared for the situation he walked into that evening. Although well intentioned, we agreed with hindsight that it had not been a good idea to ring Mum. When I calmed down I thought: what did I expect the doctor to do? Although I still think she could have been a bit more sympathetic. We needed a holiday and Dad needed a break too; we felt sure all would be okay when Mum had settled in so despite our heavy hearts we decided to stick to our holiday plans.

We caught our coach the following morning and were on our way to Austria. The first night was a sleepover in the French town of Metz. We checked in to our hotel and went out for a walk around the town. It was midsummer's day and a music festival was taking place in a small park area. We wandered freely from group to group enjoying the music and relaxing at last. We felt sure we had made the right decision and of course Mum would settle in the rest home.

We were not very late returning to our hotel as we had an early start the next morning. We entered our room, breathed a huge sigh of relief, believing we would have an undisturbed night when the telephone rang. Why in our hotel room in France was the telephone ringing? I answered it and heard a man's voice asking if he was speaking to Mrs Woolmington. "Yes," I replied, wondering why the hotel would need to speak to me. The man's reply caused me to let out an involuntary scream and hurl the receiver into the air. It was the care home calling to tell me my mother had fallen asleep in her chair that morning and passed away.

Our holiday courier was very sympathetic and helpful in arranging for Colin and I to join another coach party who had also stayed overnight at Metz on their return from Austria to the UK. So we had an emotional journey back home, poor Mum, poor Dad. How would I ever come to terms with the situation I found myself in? Guilt was threatening to engulf me. I felt better when we went to see Dad, although he did not know of my last conversation with Mum; he was obviously very upset but at least we were home and could comfort each other.

I decided to return to work and felt better for it even though I had booked the week off. Surprised colleagues asked why I wasn't on holiday and I remember telling them that my holiday was cancelled because my Mum had died. I appeared to be coping with my grief but after a few days I realised I wasn't coping at all and spent a very tearful time with the Company Personnel Officer. She was very understanding and rang my doctor there and then for an appointment. With my doctor's permission and my employers' blessing I was signed off work for as long as I needed. During that time I drove myself to Wonersh, the village of my childhood. I felt as if I had to be there even if my employers had not been understanding and it were to cost me my job I would still have gone there. I walked around the village, past Meadow View where I had grown up, along the common where I had walked with our dog Bambi, to the church where I attended Sunday school and the graveyard where Mr Hales would always kneel by his wife's grave. How empty it seemed now. I remember walking over to the grave and reading the inscription. Mr Hales was now resting with his wife.

A few months later I saw a medium on television. She was one of three being put to the test to prove their authenticity. She was referring to a Doris and a John, so of course I immediately thought of my Mum and Dad. I was impressed with this lady and wrote to the BBC enquiring how I could contact her. When I had her address I wrote asking if I could arrange to see her.

The circumstances of my mother's death still weighed on my conscience and I felt open to any route that may ease my feelings. The medium did not live locally but I arranged an appointment with her for a Sunday morning; in fact she was in the locality of Colin's parents so we combined a visit to them on the same day.

I spent an hour in the presence of this ordinary lady who had no airy-fairy ways or mumbo jumbo chants, just a lovely relaxing manner, it was just like chatting to a friend. I deliberately did not give any clues but well into our conversation when she established that she had made contact with my mother I did tell her about my fateful phone call the day before Mum died. It was an amazing experience to meet this lady and when Colin and I listened to the recording of my session with her we were both at a loss to explain how she could possibly know the things she knew. I had not given away the slightest hint of why I was there but as she held my engagement ring she told me of my mother who had passed. I had travelled to somewhere beginning and ending with the letter A, it could be America or Africa. It was Austria. She told of someone in my mother's life who died young, took their own life but not suicide. My Mum's young man had caused his accidental death when he lost control of his motorbike. She mentioned my brother and sister saying how different we all were. She also knew I had worked in London. The only thing she got wrong was that she sometimes referred to my daughter as my son, but she said my daughter would one day have a son. Just before I left she said I should love the colours of sweet peas.

I admit to a passing fascination with the spiritual world and also admit that my visit to a medium was a tremendous help to me in coming to terms with my Mum's passing. I could not alter the past but I could alter the way I coped with it. I believed Mum would not want me to feel guilty and eventually believed that the best thing I could do was to be happy – after all that's what all parents want for their children. When I arrived at work on the following Monday morning I was stunned to see a jam jar on my desk, half full of water and sweet peas. I soon realised that similar floral arrangements were on several colleagues' desks. Someone had so many in their garden they had brought them in to brighten up the workplace. Was it a co-incidence?

On my way to work one day towards the end of 1995 a white delivery van pulled away from the curb without warning, causing me to skid on the icy road and collide with a parked car I had been overtaking. Dealing with the consequential insurance claim I called in to the local office of my insurance company during December and was devastated to be told that my Fila Y10, my first car, was a write-off. Fighting back tears I returned to Colin where he was waiting for me in his car but as I got in somehow the car door swung towards me and slammed my head against the doorframe. Through my tears and pain I heard Colin say, "Well, I might as well tell you now. I've been made redundant."

It was not the best of starts to the New Year but things did get better before they got worse. My head recovered without any permanent damage (I think), I challenged the case and got my car repaired (success) and Colin found a job as a rep with one of his old company's customers (hooray).

What a blessing that our situation had improved considerably before the next blow of destiny hit us. It was the shocking tragic death of our dear friend Julie. My company granted me a compassionate day off and Colin and I joined the huge number of mourners who attended her humanitarian service.

A few years later when Dad's health and well-being was giving us concern, I was able to find a part-time job. It was no contest really, I could get another full-time job if necessary but I couldn't get another Dad. Mum and I had always been close, often chatting together while Dad did the garden or watched sport on TV. Now I had the opportunity to have chats with him. He was a lovely, genuine gentleman who had borne Mum's loss so bravely and I was glad I could spend more time with him. I remembered several years earlier when Dad's lifelong friend Harry had died. In his childhood Harry had been a Dr Barnardo's Boy and Dad often spoke emotionally of his school pal. I worried how Dad would cope with this loss but he surprised me and coped very well. Dad had been the one who sat up all night with my kitten when she had had an operation and he was the one who stood up on the top deck of a double decker bus on bonfire night and told the hooligans on board to behave themselves. He was a perfect combination of gentle and tough. He seemed so well suited to his time in service as a young man with the uniformed discipline of polite society, I think the transition to finding employment and coping with all his responsibilities of married family life must have been a quite challenge for him.

The last few years with Dad became very special, I took the opportunity to tell him what a lovely Dad he was and how much I loved him. Never one for fanciful words, but he told me I was his princess and he envied Colin getting to spend so much time with me. One thing I couldn't tell Dad was about my last talk with Mum so imagine my surprise on my visit after seeing the medium when Dad said that he had very recently felt something spiritual like the presence of Doris. I said that was a lovely thing to experience, Mum would only want to comfort him.

Having his youngest sister to stay, growing his own vegetables and enjoying games of whist were a few of the things that kept Dad busy. Even in his nineties he kept himself occupied and would often greet me with "Guess what I've done today?" If I had been in charge of Dad's village school in the early 1900s he would have been my star pupil.

When Dad had a fall in his kitchen and broke his hip I watched gratefully as the ambulance men attended and carried him out to the ambulance on a stretcher. I was reminded of the day Mum had broken her ankle in the snow and once again skilled medical men had come to our aid.

Fortunately Dad made a good recovery. He was so fascinated by the metal pin in his hip joint he arranged to have his own copy of his X-ray. This wasn't Dad's only medical misfortune. For whatever reason he was investigating between the fence and his shed in the garden when he fell and cut his hand on some large pieces of glass he had stored there. Without making a fuss he wrapped his injury in a bandage and hoped it would heal up. It did not and thankfully Dad soon realised he needed help. The state of the bungalow was evidence of the amount of blood Dad had lost, it seemed to be everywhere, so thank goodness he rang us. Another trip to hospital and another X-ray disclosed that the glass had almost sliced Dad's little finger off. The tendon was almost cut through leaving it like a frayed rope. Much to Dad's fascination he could see this by looking into the wound between his fingers. The prognosis for Dad's little finger was not good. If the wound was stitched up to heal the tendon would very likely snap if the finger was used, leaving it as a useless dangling digit that would be awkward. An operation could be done in a London hospital to fix the tendon but could mean a rigid finger that would also be awkward.

The attending doctor seemed very impressed with Dad's general lifestyle and his gardening and cooking, etc and he suggested we go and have a cup of tea for Dad to consider the best course of action for him. Initially Dad thought the operation was a good idea and I assured him it would not be a problem to go to London with him. However, after a cup of tea and further consideration he felt it would be a bit of a hassle going to London and trying to park the car, etc so maybe he would just have his wound stitched. It was a wise decision as the wound healed and Dad had no problem from his little finger.

When my daughter's wedding plans were in full swing Dad was looking forward to attending on the day. He had sorted out what he would wear including a new pair of shoes I had got for him. It was an exciting time so I think I was in denial when Dad had a mini stroke one morning when he had a problem swallowing his breakfast. It was hard to accept but Dad was taken to hospital and I had to recognize it was best for him. From now on Dad was peg fed and at one visit to see him he asked why he never got a cup of tea or food – was it because he hadn't paid?

Visiting on the seventh of September I told him it was my birthday and he apologised for not have a present for me. "No need, Dad, visiting you is enough." "That's love," he said. After my visit the next day I left the hospital, walked across the car park as usual and got in my car. Suddenly I felt like I was hit by a tidal wave, my sobs came from deep within and my tears flowed freely. It was quite a while before I composed myself enough to drive home. Early the next morning I received a telephone call from the hospital informing me that my Dad had passed away. A few weeks shy of his ninety-fourth birthday my Dad died two days after my birthday and six days before my daughter's wedding. It was a time of mixed emotions like I had never known before.

During the evening of my birthday the following year Colin and I were intrigued to hear muffled chimes from a clock in the lounge. It had been Dad's mantelpiece clock presented to him when he'd left his employment at the Astor cinema. It had an audible tick and loud chime which I had found irritating so it had never been wound up ever since it had run down. So how could we explain the continuous muffled chiming? "If it chimes seven times I'll believe it's my Dad," I said. It chimed seven times.

---oOo---

CHAPTER IX

Rod and Julie
or
the house called Sea View

My daughter had her first introduction to swimming when she was six months old. As I held her, dressed only in a nappy, and dipped her gently into the sea as the waves rolled in, she loved it and squealed with delight. When she was a little older it was always a pleasure to take her to a sports centre swimming pool, something we did most weeks. Supported by her inflated red armbands and supervised by Colin, who didn't swim, she would bob around happily in the shallow end, while I could enjoy a good exercise session, swimming lengths. So, for quite some time, we all enjoyed our regular visits to the pool, until Katherine began to float independently and venture into deeper water. This was great for our daughter, and although we were delighted with her progress, which we had encouraged, it was a bit sad for her Dad whose role was now redundant and frustrating for me because it was now virtually impossible to swim an uninterrupted length of the pool. The only solution was for all of us to be able to swim. Colin said he would learn, but when?

The following Christmas I enrolled Colin for swimming lessons at our local sports centre, as part of his Christmas present. He wasn't too excited; in fact, he was somewhat indignant. He would have swimming lessons when he was ready, in his own time. No way did he need or want his life organised for him! Okay, I had enrolled him in the classes, but that didn't mean he had to attend! The subject was not for discussion and the start of term was fast approaching. On the day of the first lesson, Colin went out with his cossi and towel. Would he attend the classes, I wondered – yes he did. I can't say he took to swimming like a duck to water but he continued to attend regularly. The fact that he had become quite pally with another learner made it all the more bearable. Advancement was slow, Colin was finding it difficult to take his feet off the bottom of the pool and trust that his body could be suspended in water without sinking. Then there was a turning point, one week the usual coach was away and a lady instructor took the class. Suddenly Colin could take his feet off the bottom and stay afloat in deeper water, for the first time.

Along with his swimming ability, Colin was definitely making a new friend with the fellow beginner called Rod. He and Rod decided that their new skill would benefit from some practice in between the lessons. Rod's partner called Julie was a keen swimmer so we made a foursome on Saturday mornings and had extra-curricular swimming sessions. This proved to be brilliant fun, as it was never very busy and quite often we virtually had the pool to ourselves. So grew a really good friendship.

Rod and Julie were much younger than us, we could just about have been their parents; in fact Julie was just eighteen days old on the day we got married. They were also quite different characters from most of our friends. I recall popping round to see them one day to discover Rod at home on his own, Julie was down the road with her head under the bonnet, where her car had broken down. He made us a cup of tea and settled down for a chat. Had that been our predicament,

Colin would be fixing the car and I would be making the tea. Rod was a professional keyboard player, who started his career as one half of a musical duo called Eye to Eye. He now worked with a partner, making the type of music used as background music for supermarkets and adverts. Every few weeks he would don his one and only dinner suit, white shirt and red bow tie and play a grand piano in the large foyer of a swish hotel in Bracknell. What a coincidence when some friends of ours arranged to have their daughter's wedding reception at the very hotel and the date coincided with Rod's piano playing booking. We attended the wedding and saw our slim, young friend providing beautiful background music for all the guests. We hardly recognised him in his best togs!

Rod drove a vintage white Mercedes with a sound system creating all-round-wrap-around music to envelope the senses. Whenever he drove us anywhere I always reckoned I could take up residence and live in his car.

Julie was a bit of a tomboy. She bombed around in a burgundy coloured MG Midget and worked as a building inspector for Slough Council. She didn't wear makeup or jewellery, didn't own a handbag, and dressed in t-shirt and jogging bottoms. She once told us about her frock, the only one she had owned in her adult life. It was purchased for a work's do, worn once and ended its days as a wearable garment when Rod introduced it to the wrong washing machine programme. It was never replaced.

Julie was a one-off, independent, interesting and funny but not outrageous. Much less demonstrative than Rod, Julie had a musical side too. Although, according to Colin on our wedding day, I sang flat and did not have an ear for music, I loved listening to the guitar, so one Christmas he generously, or misguidedly, bought me a guitar. Needless to say, I never mastered playing it although I did try. I even made the huge sacrifice of cutting my fingernails really short, showing just how seriously I was trying. One day at our house, Julie started strumming my guitar and unfortunately one of the strings broke. On her next visit she replaced the guitar's metal strings with nylon ones, tuned the instrument and proceeded to sing a song to Colin. This proved to be one of our abiding memories of our special friend Julie.

Something really gelled between the four of us and we became firm friends. Our Saturday swimming sessions extended to lunch together, initially at a local tea shop then, as our friendship grew, alternating between their place and ours and invariably lunchtime extended well into the afternoon. Such easy company, we could just sit and chat effortlessly for hours. They were a very genuine, unpretentious couple and even now, I often quote one of my favourite lines Rod said whilst eating bread and jam at our place: "I'm having a lovely time".

They shared their semi-detached house in the middle of Guildford with their black and white cat. Their house was called "Sea View" and the cat was called "Cat". Obviously! Rod and Julie's house had a cellar, which they had converted into a studio for playing and recording music. It was as fascinating for us to see all of Rod's high tech equipment as it was amusing for him to see all our 45 rpm records and turntable. He very kindly offered to record some of our records onto tape for us and so we enjoyed several nostalgic recording sessions in his cellar, for which we are eternally grateful.

Winter evenings at their place were very relaxed and cosy, sitting and chatting, by the fire. It was even cosier one year when Rod proudly installed his latest purchase: a six foot tall Christmas tree, which virtually took over their lounge!

Compared to us with my organised holiday planning, Rod and Julie were reckless globetrotters, their next destination often being the result of sticking a pin in the atlas. To say they travelled light was a bit of an understatement – as long as they had PMT (passport, money and tickets), they were ready for the off!

Whereas I would buy new clothes for my trip, they preferred to shop as they travelled. I remember taking Rod to task one day about the state of the footwear he proposed travelling in. We duly received a postcard they sent from Hong Kong: "Old trainers dumped in bin, new ones purchased!" They enjoyed visiting exotic places like Mexico, Thailand or South America, often saying they would love to sell up and go to live in Brazil. They did have a Brazilian friend called Merris, with a boyfriend called Maurice, who owned some land in Brazil. It was their daydream to have their home built out there.

Much to the amusement of Rod and Julie, most of our holidays were spent in our touring caravan and often our conversations were travel based. So it was no surprise that we came round to discussing going away together. They had never camped before and despite Rod's genuine trepidation, they were persuaded to embark on a weekend away with us. We towed our caravan and they followed, with a borrowed tent, in Julie's MG Midget. We chose a picturesque site in Devon, near an old mill with a stream running close by. It was idyllic.

Arriving early in the evening we had plenty of time to set up camp before sunset. Julie set to erecting their tent while Rod chatted with us and got used to his surroundings. So far so good, we all enjoyed supper in our caravan before bidding each other goodnight. Rod and Julie trotted off to their tent and we made up our bed to settle down for the night. I adored our caravan, to me it was like playing house, and it was exciting to be sharing this weekend with our good friends Rod and Julie.

Not long after snuggling into our cosy sleeping bags we heard the familiar drumming of rain on our caravan roof. Thank goodness it had held off until the night, we said, and not spoilt our day. So, to the sound of raindrops falling on our roof, we drifted off to sleep, blissfully unaware that the rainfall was getting heavier and heavier.

It was in the very early hours of the morning that we were awakened by urgent knocking on our caravan door. Colin jumped out of bed and opened the door to investigate. It was still raining and our friends were standing on our threshold. I jumped out of bed too, to see what was happening and promptly wished I hadn't. The sight of me in a dry, lit, cosy caravan dressed in cream silk pyjamas was almost too much to bear for our cold, damp, dishevelled friends who had not slept a wink but lain wide awake in their dark, cold, leaking tent.

Despite our offering a shelter for the night, albeit very cramped, in our caravan, they insisted they would not disturb us further but would be grateful if they could have our keys so they could spend the rest of the night in our car. There was nothing to be gained by prolonging the discussion in those conditions at that time of night, so we gave them the keys. They disappeared into the darkness and we got back into our luxury, high tog sleeping bags. Could we sleep? No! We wrestled with our conscience, fretted and felt guilty about our friends' plight until eventually Colin decided the least we could do was make them a hot cup of tea. The kettle was boiled, the tea was made and delivered to the occupants of our car. Gratitude was somewhat strained as Colin's knocking on the car window roused them from a slumber they had just managed to achieve.

Of course our friendship survived, it even flourished. Further holiday discussions with Rod and Julie focused on a different mode of transport, warmer climes and a different choice of accommodation. So it was that we all flew to Spain and stayed for a week in a one bedroom apartment in Denya, owned by our other lovely friends Pat and Pete – yet another test for our friendship. Despite Colin's fear of flying and our lack of globetrotting experience we set off without any misgivings. There was no dispute over the accommodation: not only were we the seniors, we were married. We had the bedroom and Rod and Julie slept on the sofa bed in the lounge. It really was a great holiday with lots of good memories. Rod and Julie hired scooters one day while we cautiously hired pushbikes. They obviously explored further afield than us but at least we didn't have any mishaps like Rod did. Luckily nothing was broken but lots of TLC required for his cuts and grazes.

We had a wonderful day when we drove up through the mountains in our hire car, soaking up the fantastic scenery. We made lots of stops on our tour, for photo opportunities, until we realised we were very hungry, miles from anywhere and it was almost siesta time. To our relief, a small cluster of buildings including a café came into view. We parked the car and approached anxiously, would they be open? It transpired that the café owners were about to tuck into their plates of paella, which they had just put on the table. We managed to explain that we were hoping to buy ourselves some food and they responded in typical Spanish style; with much flourishing of arms and smiles they whisked their plates to the back of the café and served their starving tourists with plates of paella!

On the return leg of our journey, again in a remote area, we stopped at a garage. We left discussions completely to Rod and Julie this time while we waited in the car. After quite some time, they returned and appeared to be quite excited about something. They had recognised the artist, whose guitar music had been playing in the garage, as someone they knew. They learned from the garage proprietor that the musician had suffered an accident and lost the use of his right arm. He had subsequently taught himself to play his guitar left handed, and now lived in Spain.

It wasn't high summer during our stay, but it was certainly warm enough to sit in the sun by the swimming pool, catching up with some holiday reading. At least, two of us did – I had my knitting and Colin paced about, testing the water and trying to drum up some enthusiasm for a swim al fresco. No amount of bullying would persuade Rod or Julie to even dip their toes in the water so eventually

I gave in and joined Colin in the pool – it was freezing. I remember it so clearly and the date was 5 November!

Not long after our return home, Rod and Julie presented us with an amazing memento of our Spanish adventure. Our talented friends had made a recording of their version of 'Don't Put Your Daughter on the Stage, Mrs Worthington', entitled 'Don't Put Your Husband on the Plane, Mrs Woolmington'. Although the humorous lyrics were at our expense, it was brilliant.

For many years Colin and I had been active supporters of the Guildford School of Acting and we frequently encouraged friends and work colleagues to make up a party booking to see the students' productions. In this way, several of our friends became acquainted with more of our friends. So it was that Rod and Julie met and got on very well with our good friends John and Hilary. We decided it would be rather good to have an evening all together so we invited them round to ours for a meal. My social conscience getting the better of me, I will admit to suggesting to John and Hilary that they dress down for the occasion, as Rod and Julie were always casually dressed. It makes me blush to think of it now as they were the least likely people I know to feel uncomfortable about what they were wearing. Come the night, I dressed down and I was the one to answer the doorbell. Our friends all arrived together, both men dressed in dinner jackets and bow ties! Can't one even trust one's friends?

It was well into our friendship when we learned that Julie was a Samaritan. In my late teens another of my friends had also been a Samaritan and I really wanted to be one myself. What an amazing organisation and what a comfort to know there was always someone there for anyone in distress, any time of the day or night. Marriage, full time work and our full social life were all contributing factors to why I did not join up, but I held it in my mind, for the future.

When the Samaritans held a Summer Fete just outside Guildford, Rod and Julie were obviously involved in the event. As well as the usual fete stalls the main attraction was duck racing. Each duck was identified by a coloured bow round its neck and bets were placed on the duck of your choice. Julie had an idea for another fundraising stall with a difference: a human fruit machine. All she needed was a couple of willing, gullible volunteers to help run it. You've guessed it – we were roped in as part of the team. Three chairs were placed in line, and screened off with a windbreaker, so each occupant could not see the others. A chart portraying the value of two bananas or three lemons, etc was displayed and the three of us each occupied a chair and held a bag containing five fruits: an apple, an orange, a lemon, a kiwi fruit, and a banana. The punters paid their money and at the given signal, Julie, Colin and I produced a fruit from our bag. According to the chart, they either won some money back or lost the lot. It was brilliant and great fun, even if it did get a bit messy by the end of the day – bananas and kiwi fruit did not respond well to constant handling.

When Colin's boss, at the time, invited us to a company bash, in the guise of a St Trinian's Party, it was Julie's turn to help me out with my costume. All my school clothes, including my tie, were long gone but Julie still had lots of hers. I borrowed her short pleated netball skirt, her school tie, hat and satchel. I completed the ensemble with a white shirt, deliberately laddered black stockings my hair in bunches and my cheeks dotted with freckles. Although I say it myself, I looked every inch of a St Trinian's girl. However, Colin outshone me with his Headmaster's get-up. Stick-on side whiskers, moustache and a swishy cane gave him the winning edge and he won first prize for the best fancy dress costume.

We all seemed to be mutually enjoying all the extra social time together and our regular Saturday morning swimming sessions continued. It was hard to accept the news when Rod and Julie explained that they were having difficulties in their relationship. It was 1995 and the Bosnian war was raging. A young man who had been connected with the Guildford School of Acting, had been instrumental in setting up a charity called Phoenix Aid and Julie had become passionate about joining the charity. Indeed, there had been a meeting in a church hall in Guildford, held to raise awareness of the plight of the civilians caught up in the war. We showed support for our friend by attending the meeting with her and Rod.

We were still good friends, but there developed a slight strain in our meetings. Conversation would often focus on the ugliness of war and unjust treatment of innocent people. Of course, we all held the same views on the subject but it seemed to be having a negative effect on Rod and Julie's relationship. The more Julie felt compelled to act on her feelings, the more nervous Rod became of losing her. It was a sensitive, somewhat scary time, for them. Their affection for each other was obvious – they had not needed to be demonstrative about it but I recall how they held hands and walked on their own a lot and even embraced as we walked from the swimming pool one Saturday morning.

Shortly after this Julie joined Phoenix Aid on a six week working party in Bosnia. On her return, she visited us, without Rod. It was a poignant evening spent together, it felt as if time with our special friend was finite and very precious. Julie's time in a war zone hadn't really changed her priorities and outlook on life; it had endorsed all that she believed in and brought it into sharp focus. She was, and still is, the least materialistic person I have ever known. She told me how she had walked in Guildford full of shops, full of Christmas things and all the people buying things and all she could think of was the Bosnian mud still on her boots and what it represented. She talked of the Bosnian situation and how people's lives were affected by the war. Whilst I understood and shared her compassion I struggled with the extent of her commitment to leave the security of her home, her job, her partner, her family and her country. However, that is exactly what she did.

Colin and I felt a pride in knowing Julie and what she was planning to do but also great sadness that she was going away and a fear for her safety. When she moved out of her home with Rod, left her job and spent all her money on a white Land Rover, we knew there was no turning back, she was on her way.

We were pleased to be able to correspond with Julie; somehow our letters got through to her, as did a large jar of Marmite we optimistically posted off to her – she loved it! In one of her long letters to us she related how she had driven her Land Rover over the mountains to reunite her refugee passengers with their family for Christmas. Despite the hazardous conditions, not to mention there being a war on, and the police border controls and security guards that she had to contend with, she made it through to achieve her goal. That was the Julie we knew; we'd have been surprised if she hadn't made it. She wrote that no amount of Christmas shopping could compare with the joy of that family's reunion – it was the best Christmas present ever. Yes, now I fully understood her cynical view of materialism and what it meant to her to have Bosnian mud on her boots.

I was listening to the Archers on the radio whilst preparing our meal one evening when a phone call from our friend Hilary interrupted me. A report on the television news related how a young woman, volunteering for Phoenix Aid in Bosnia, had been killed. It was Julie. I don't remember whether we ate our meal but I know I certainly never heard the end of the Archers. We knew that two young men, working for the same charity, had recently been killed and now, the unspeakable fear we had felt had happened. Julie had been driving in a convoy of lorries delivering coal and other goods to a school, when her vehicle veered off the road and overturned as it rolled down a bank.

Julie was young enough to be my daughter and yet, during our friendship, she had taught me so much about life. She made me start to rethink a lot of my fixed ideas, question some of my values and take a broader view on things. Julie was an amazing friend who had the confidence and courage of her conviction. It was a great privilege to have known her. I knew I was far from alone in this privilege, for her humanitarian service was attended by the largest attendance I have ever seen at a funeral.

Her photograph on a memorial stone on a roadside in Bosnia marks the place where Julie died, at the age of 39. A memorial plaque in the National Memorial Arboretum in Alrewas, Staffordshire reads: "Planted for Julie J Morrant 1 December 1964 - 16 January 1996 who lost her life in Bosnia helping to relieve the suffering of the people there. Her laughter and determination are forever in our thoughts".

Julie enriched the lives of those who knew her and we were fortunate to be included.

Sea View in Guildford was sold and Rod moved nearer to London. Our friendship continued and we spent many a lovely musical evening at Rod's place with his interesting friends. It always finished up with Rod giving us all the benefit of his talent on the keyboard. Rod learned and became fluent in Portuguese and after his mother died, he sold his property and went to live in the sunshine in Brazil.

---oOo---

CHAPTER X

My story

At the dawn of the 21st century, in 2000, I started work in my last job before retirement which proved to have very flexible working hours providing I did my thirty hours a week. At the time I didn't know that histopathology was the study of diseased tissue but it sounded interesting so when I spotted an advert for a part-time secretary at a local medical practice I applied and got the job. Colin and I did our sums and took a calculated risk when Colin took early retirement. I continued in my job and negotiated a five-week break, enabling us to take a fantastic trip to New Zealand. We toured north and south island by hire car and stayed in motels. It was also wonderful to be able to visit friends who had taken up residence there and worked for New Zealand Light Leather following the closure of Gomshall Tannery. Despite the twenty-four hour journey we both hoped that another visit might be possible one day.

In 2005 I reached my official retirement age of sixty but I worked on for a further eighteen months as my job was due to finish then anyway. This was not a problem at all as it was part-time employment and I enjoyed it. However, given that choice now, I know I would never again sacrifice a single day of my retirement; time is far too precious.

I had often hoped to move to a smaller more conveniently located residence when we retired even though I dreaded having to leave our house with so many good memories. A second wonderful trip to New Zealand straight after my retirement added to this dilemma. In Geraldine, a small South Island town where we felt very much at home we were moved to view a few properties, and I found my dream home. A similar property in the UK in our area would be beyond our reach financially. I thought the detached bungalow with its gravel drive, pretty veranda and garage/sleepover in the garden was perfect for us in our retirement. Its location was almost perfect too, within walking distance of the small town and there was even a golf club at the end of the road for Colin. Why was it so far away on the other side of the world? It made me feel unsettled.

Just like everyone else my life had its ups and downs but we had weathered the storms of two redundancies and coped with the loss of our parents plus all the other everyday problems along the way. Why, now, had I started to become a serious worrier? I hadn't sailed through life without a care in the world, but this was different. Anxiety and panic attacks started to plague me.

I pushed the lever as usual but didn't get the usual response. I pushed it again, still no response. I pushed again then again, still no reassuring gurgling of water flushing the loo. What do I do now? Call a plumber of course. Why didn't Colin agree with me? Didn't he appreciate the seriousness and urgency of the situation? The toilet cistern was not working, it might malfunction and flood the house, and we could drown in our bed. Just because it was nearly midnight, it didn't seem a good enough reason not to call a plumber without delay. This situation had to be dealt with and dealt with NOW! Why couldn't Colin see the urgency of the situation? It couldn't wait until morning; it seemed like a matter of life or death to me!

This wasn't the first time I felt frustrated and misunderstood lately and it seemed to be happening more and more. Just like it was with the garden, nobody took me seriously when I worried about being able to cope with weed control in our large garden. I never really enjoyed gardening and only did it because I liked to see it tidy. The size of our garden had always overwhelmed me and now, in my mind, it was becoming the size of a huge jungle, and the plants were threatening to take over, covering the windows and enveloping the whole house. I had visions of the house being swathed in wild greenery and the roof disappearing under trails of ivy. If we were indoors we wouldn't be able to get out and if we were outside we wouldn't be able to get in. Where would we live? What would become of us?

Everything seemed to be getting ridiculous and distorted and everything was getting out of proportion. I was struggling to understand why nobody shared my point of view and the mental conflict in my brain was becoming overwhelming. How could everyone carry on with their lives without sharing my concern about all these serious things? Why did I feel like I was swimming against the tide, out of step with life and constantly losing ground?

I had sought my doctor's help quite early on. He seemed sympathetic, and told me of people who had suffered depression and even gone missing but had come through it and recovered. I completed his questionnaire and one of the questions it asked was 'Had I considered self-harming?' I considered this thoughtfully and answered 'No'. I had become a manic mess of panic, completely devoid of pleasure, and in constant pain. Harming myself would be the last thing I would think of doing, surely adding to my hurt; I didn't need *that*, I needed something to *stop* my pain.

The diagnosis for me was clinical depression with classic symptoms of anxiety and for many weeks I swallowed the prescribed daily dose of antidepressants, waiting for a glimmer of hope to shine in my blackness. It didn't happen, my living hell and my panic attacks continued. I rang the surgery one day, almost screaming to talk to my doctor. He was not available but another doctor came to the phone. I remember standing in my kitchen holding the phone to my ear while being instructed to take deep breaths or breathe into a paper bag. "I've done all that," I shouted back, completely out of character for me, "it doesn't work!" What a doctor's dilemma! I'm not sure whether I could cope with a completely hysterical female on the phone, but then, I haven't had the training.

Shortly after this episode I had a home visit from my doctor. We sat at the kitchen table and talked while he tried to reassure me. Even though I listened, desperately wanting his words to help, nothing comforted me. I reached out and seized his hand, pleading for him to help me. I was too scared to tell my husband or family, my doctor or my friends exactly what my mind was making me think. I was too scared to even believe it myself. I desperately needed someone to talk to, someone I could truthfully tell all about my state of mind. In all my life, I swear I had never known such despair. Even the pain I felt when I lost my parents could not begin to match this agony; it was completely alien.

However radical a change is, when it begins small and grows very gradually, it is often difficult to realise the change that is happening and hard to remember how or when it started. So it was with my depression. How would I or anyone else know that my lack of enthusiasm to do anything wasn't just a 'down' day, a bad hair day or even the start of a cold? I do not know when my desire to stay in and not see friends turned into a fear of socialising and a terror of getting lost in the big frightening world. When did the pleasure of shopping or lunching with friends become an unbearable crushing challenge?

I knew I was not good company and lots of friends went to great lengths to try and cheer me up but despite their valiant efforts, nothing worked. A shopping trip to Kingston by bus with a friend, and having free travel with our senior citizens' bus passes, was something I would have previously jumped at excitedly but now it was a huge ordeal. The journey seemed endless and I felt scared all the time. We had lunch in John Lewis; how I remember the agony of having to choose something to eat. I was so frightened of getting lost, when my friend momentarily disappeared from my field of vision in the shoe department, a big wave of panic washed over me.

I became very frugal to the point of meanness when using household products. I had to preserve our stock of everything from toothpaste to washing up liquid. I could not contemplate running out of anything because that would mean having to go shopping. I remember a supermarket trip where I spent the whole time worrying about using my credit card in case I wasn't around to settle the account and that would be another problem for Colin.

Colin tried many things to make me feel better. He took me for cycle rides, one of my favourite pursuits but all to no avail. We cycled to a garden centre one Sunday and had a cup of tea in their café. Horror of horrors, there was someone there who I knew. She saw me and asked how I was. My feeble attempt to appear relaxed and "fine thanks" was excruciating for me. I hated watching other people going about their business, meeting friends, eating out and enjoying life. How could they do that when I was suffering, it was so unfair. Sadly, I had no appetite or energy for anything, anywhere at any time and I knew that someone who cannot be cheered up is no fun at all. What was the point?

If I had broken a leg or arm or been diagnosed with a physical illness, of course, it would have been a very different scenario. Everyone would know what was wrong with me, know what to say and know what to focus on. No one actually mentioned mental illness. I guess all the fearful implications associated with it made it too frightening to identify it audibly although I guess that's what they were all thinking.

I could not talk to anyone about my fear and yet I felt desperate for someone to talk to. I was petrified of being alone, and yet felt so alone all the time. What hope was there when my own mind contradicted itself? Lots of things were changing, life was getting distorted and I could neither hide it nor explain it and I hated it.

All my personal worries had become overwhelmingly and completely out of proportion, life was completely devoid of any pleasure, only a growing panic and fear. I was literally begging for counselling and eventually I received a letter from the NHS Foundation Trust, Primary Care Mental Health Service. Was I on my way to salvation? Not yet, I was on a waiting list! I still have that letter in my file. Dated 23 May 2008, written at least three weeks after my referral, it stated:

"We are a small service and receive a high volume of referrals. As a result we are unable to offer you an immediate appointment. The current waiting time is approximately 16 to 20 weeks. When we are able to see you for an assessment we will contact you with an appointment.

Please note that we are not able to offer urgent appointments and would advise you to return to your GP to discuss other options for support if you require immediate help.

If you would require any further information about our service then please contact us."

A sixteen to twenty week wait! It seemed cruel and unbelievably shocking. Did I have what it took to wait that long? To me this seemed only to illustrate the ignorance or apathy of the system when it came to mental health issues. Whatever one's problem the sooner help is forthcoming the better; waiting only prolongs the agony.

Nevertheless, I can now think of a possible couple of things in defence of the system: an obvious lack of sufficient resources and the ability of the patient to disguise the severity of their affliction. I believe the latter would be managed out of fear of the consequences of being thought mad and possibly sectioned in a mental hospital and also the stigma associated with mental illness. I was lucky in that I was retired, I can't imagine the exaggerated state of anxiety and stress for someone trying to cope with the added pressure of maintaining employment. Fear is a powerful silencer. Many things are fearful but none more so than the prospect of losing your mind or being deprived of your freedom.

I stopped watching television because I could not tolerate watching fictional programmes that I couldn't even concentrate on. It just seemed like such a waste of time but I didn't want to do anything else either, it was madness. My beloved Radio 4, which used to entertain me throughout the day, also seemed pointless. Newspapers were full of horror stories of financial crises and banks crashing, wars being fought, people committing suicide, it was horrendous, the world was definitely going mad. Simple mental tasks were beyond me – I couldn't even do the easy crossword anymore or compete with Colin, as we had always done, doing the word game from the newspaper. He usually got more words than me but to his indignation, his victory was often disputed, some of his words were decidedly suspect! Although I tried to make words out of the given letters, my brain seemed incapable of spelling anything and this inability just made me more frightened and fearful of the future.

I dreaded the post coming through the letterbox, it would probably mean having to deal with something, I don't know what I thought would arrive. As for computers and mobile phones – they terrified me; I felt embarrassed that I couldn't begin to understand how to operate them.

All the everyday inconveniences of life had become big problems to me, way out of proportion. I imagined my head was like a big, grey, metal water tank. Every problem was a bubble pushing and squashing its way into the tank but my biggest problem was that the tank was getting too full. There wasn't room for any more bubbles but they kept coming and the tank was overflowing – I was literally suffocating in the bubbles. Sometimes even breathing was a challenge.

Daytime was becoming unbearable. I longed for bedtime when I could at least legitimately switch off from the world and retreat to my own private planet. My sleep, when it came, was short lived. I would just lie in the dark, wondering where the person I used to be had gone. I remember, on just one occasion, actually lying awake for the entire night. I told my doctor I was not sleeping and for the first, and so far the only time in my life, I had sleeping pills. With hindsight I wonder now whether my need for sleeping pills should have been more deeply explored before being prescribed. My anxiety state was recognized – should more questions have been asked? However, I obtained my prescribed sleeping pills and within a short time of taking one I was fast asleep, like magic. Exactly two hours later I was awake again. What good was that? I didn't feel like I had slept at all, it was just two hours later than when I took the pill. When the dreaded pale light of dawn crept through the curtains I knew the hell would start again and, without a real break from it, I would have to face another twenty-four hours. An added nightmare was the dawn chorus, that incessant bird song welcoming the new day. Didn't they know I didn't welcome it? Why did they have to torture me so? Couldn't they put it on hold while I was suffering and give me some peace? In truth, I don't think it would have made any difference; I'm sure I would have just carried on suffering in silence! My distress was so intense.

Food was becoming an increasing problem. Whether it was sweet or savoury it did not seem to matter, it all tasted of nothing. I couldn't even eat in the privacy of my own home; somehow food formed itself into what seemed like a ball of cotton wool in my dry mouth and was impossible to swallow. My saliva glands seemed to have stopped functioning, I could seldom swallow anything. I could drink water and tea but developed an aversion to coffee. Goodness knows what I thought would happen if I drank coffee, I never found out, I was too frightened to try. I started to lose weight so had to select clothes to try and disguise the fact.

My panic was affecting me physically and emotionally, inside and out, it was all consuming. My hands and feet were always moist with perspiration, I couldn't write anything down as my damp hand would affect the paper and the pen wouldn't write. The pitch of my voice had changed so that I sounded very tight and harsh and I couldn't do anything to relax my throat muscles and sound normal again. If I answered the phone the caller always asked if it was Colin – I stopped wanting to talk to anyone. What the hell was happening? Was I turning into someone else?

We heard from our dear friend Rod, who had sold up and moved to Rio de Janeiro; he was visiting the UK and would like to come and see us. I had missed our friend very much and should have been thrilled at the prospect of his visit but I couldn't begin to think about coping and catering for a visitor, I just panicked. NO WAY. What was wrong with me? Rod was the absolute easiest of guests. It still saddens me to know that we missed his visit. Why on earth did I worry about catering? Rod would have been happy eating bread and jam.

The fear I experienced while my life seemed to be disintegrating manifested itself in a hollow kind of ache in the pit of my stomach. It churned my guts, agitated my mind and tortured my very being. I was powerless to control it and yet it had the power to control me. Sometimes the burning feeling in my chest was like a ball of fire and the pain would spread down my arms, like an inferno consuming my muscles and overriding my brain signals to my limbs. My arms felt numb and weak – was I suffering a form of paralysis? At my worst moments my legs weakened too, adding to my panic: would I become unable to walk? I began to wonder just how much more of this I could take.

All I wanted was 'out' so no one would have to worry about me anymore. Surely if I wasn't here there would be nothing to worry about. By this time I had decided it was unbearable to go on giving my family and friends so much worry; the only way to ease their concern and my agonising pain was not to be here; that would end everyone's problem. No way could I continue waiting for a counsellor, I felt like I was going insane, it was unbearable, I had to get out, so I allowed fanciful thoughts of leaving the planet to enter my mind. Just thinking about it seemed a huge distraction from my agony – if no one else could understand or help me then the solution was obvious: I had to help myself. On top of my own suffering, the worry and distress I knew I was causing my family and friends was placing an unbearable burden of guilt on me. At that time I believed suicide was the only way to stop my suffering, all I had to do was decide how. Admitting this fact is excruciatingly demanding to do but I believe in the need to do so. Now it is benignly painful in comparison to when I was suffering.

Dear Colin, he must have been feeling quite at a loss to know what to do with his problem wife. He also took me for walks in our favourite haunts where we used to go when we were courting. We parked the car one day and followed the familiar footpath past the old mill at Shalford, to the Chantries, a beautiful area of wooded hills with distant views over Guildford, Pewley Downs and St Martha's Church at Chilworth beyond. I clearly remember standing in a grassy clearing surrounded by beautiful, tall evergreen trees and seeing Guildford Cathedral at a distance almost level with us on Stag Hill. Colin held me safely in his arms and gently asked me to tell him what was troubling me. That moment was the closest I came to telling him that I just could not bear my life anymore. But when I looked at his face I could not say anything, I didn't know what was wrong with me and I was franticly trying to find a way to put it right. If I told him what I was thinking about it would surely upset him and it would probably be the end of any plan of mine; I could not risk that.

At last, I finally, fully realised something, it felt almost as though I had come to my senses. Of course, if nobody can help me then I would have to find my own way out and help myself. From then on my mind could think of nothing but trying to find a way out of the hell I was in. I knew everyone was worried about me and I knew I had to put a stop to their worry and my torment. Although, in some ways, it was a negative line of thought it seemed something very positive to me, a bit of a relief, something for me to concentrate on. When executed, my solution would bring me peace forever and that was very appealing.

At last I felt I was gaining some kind of control, I had a plan to focus on and it was a welcome relief. Even better than that, my plan had several plots and I could fill many hours of my incessant days and nights absorbed in the endless feasibilities, possibilities and practicalities of my plan. I had to put an end to everyone's worry and my living hell.

My hell ended on the 7 July 2008.

In my hospital bed I read a letter Colin brought to me. It was a copy of a second letter from the NHS Foundation Trust, Primary Care Mental Health Service to my doctor which made reference to my referral in April 2008 for help with depression and stress management and confirms that I was offered an appointment for an assessment in August 2008. However, I was unable to keep the appointment owing to ongoing hospital treatment following a serious accident. If it wasn't so tragic it would be funny!

Even though I now have personal experience of suffering severe depression, I certainly would not profess to have all the answers for a fellow sufferer. However, in my book, appropriate professional help is the only route to starting to find a cure and the sooner the better.

In September 2014 a headline from the Independent stated that since 2012 "Thousands attempt suicide while on NHS waiting list for psychological help". I felt lessons needed to be learned. I recently checked my local Waverley Community Mental Health Recovery

Service on the internet and was amazed and relieved to read that waiting lists are currently twenty-eight days for routine appointments, five days for urgent appointments and emergency referrals will be assessed on the same day. Could this really be true? I was also impressed to read the very comprehensive information regarding their contact, services and referral system. What a huge relief to read all this – I hardly dare believe it. To double check I rang the Service and had it verbally confirmed that it was true. It would appear that lessons have been learned.

I have also asked my doctor about the questionnaire he had asked me to complete. He showed me the current version of it, including a question about wanting to die or self-harm. Although it could not be confirmed I felt sure the questionnaire had been updated and quite rightly so. I'm pretty sure I remember the original wording of that particular question correctly and there was no mention of suicidal thoughts.

I can believe that my doctor may not have been greatly experienced in dealing with mental illness and he was doing his best for me given the limitations of the services available. I also believe it is an appalling state of affairs that the services available were so inadequate when figures being produced show that mental illness is a rapidly increasing problem.

When I recently learned that patients can now self-refer, I decided to find out more about it. I read about Improving Access to Psychological Therapies (IAPT) which is an NHS initiative designed to make psychological or talking therapies more accessible to people experiencing common mental health problems. The talking therapies offered were approved by the National Institute for Health and Care Excellence (NICE) which meant that they were proven to be effective treatments for problems such as depression and anxiety.

Then I read that there are exclusions to the self-referral route: Amongst others, it does not work for people who have complex difficulties such as personality disorder or are at risk of self-harm or suicide; or have a history of abuse issues where this would be the focus of treatment. Further reading informed me that if there was imminent risk of harm to oneself or to someone else IAPT were duty bound to inform another professional. But I've just read that it is does not work for anyone at risk of self-harm or suicide so I would not have gone ahead with self-referral.

I had the privilege to tell my story at a women's prison and during a question and answer session following my talk it was unanimously agreed that fear was the main factor for not being able to admit how one truly felt. If fear stops a clinically depressed person admitting the true depth of their anxiety, I doubt there would be a chance of them actually writing it down to complete a self-referral form. I think it is reasonable to believe that many would rather find an alternative way to end their suffering than admit it in writing. Just as well I was not offered self-referral; it would not have worked for me. Sadly, many people suffering like I did must slip through the net.

Thankfully the stigma of mental illness is becoming less of a burden nowadays. Many celebrities talk openly about it, many books are published about it and high profile people including royalty are raising awareness. I believe all this helps tremendously. Is it possible, I wonder, for a non-sufferer to fully appreciate the white-hot fear and pain of severe clinical depression?

Everybody has problems and worries but not everybody suffers depression. I don't think it is the size or quantity of problems that makes people mentally ill, it is the way they deal with them. Some people see travelling by aeroplane as an exciting adventure whilst others are so stressed by the prospect they require medication to be able to cope. There are many different reasons for wanting to end one's life and each reason has its own symptoms. In my case I had a complete loss of pleasure in life. I felt depressed, anxious and hopeless and had lost abilities I used to have to solve problems, undertake tasks or make decisions. I felt a burden to others and had no role in society.

It is a fact that there have been cultures in the world where rational or altruistic suicide is seen as an act of respect, courage and wisdom. Maybe if I had belonged to such a culture, I would not have had any shame or embarrassment to deal with.

It is well to remember that mental illness does not discriminate amongst its victims. No amount of riches, education, status or location can protect anyone; nor can a total lack of these things: depression can happen to anyone.

--oOo--

CHAPTER XI

In hospital

It was a Monday morning in July when I apparently told Colin I needed some things for our holiday on the Isles of Scilly in a few days' time and intended to walk into town for my shopping. This must have seemed incredibly calm and organised, considering the state I had been in for the previous few months and no doubt Colin felt quite encouraged about my condition, thinking I was looking forward to our holiday. We had been visiting the beautiful, 'fortunate' isles annually for many years, always booking at the end of each holiday for the following year. I had even started getting things out and ready for packing.

It would seem that as I walked along the main road into town a neighbour drove by the other way. He waved to me but I completely ignored him. As far I was concerned, I didn't even know I was walking into town, let alone see a neighbour wave to me.

Neither did I have the slightest recollection of the previous day when a very good friend came round to watch the televised men's Wimbledon final tennis match with us. Roger Federer and Rafael Nadal fought it out in a match lasting four hours and forty-eight minutes, the third longest men's singles final in history. An epic tournament, heralded as one of the greatest matches in the history of tennis. When I was told this I denied all knowledge of it and was very annoyed that I had missed the match.

Before Colin could start to worry that I had been too long in town, he heard the doorbell ring. There on the doorstep were two policemen, undisputable evidence that all was not well. I find it unbearably painful to imagine the scene, as Colin was told that I had had a very serious, life threatening accident and was in hospital in London. Naturally he wanted to be with me, and unfortunately the officers were not able to accompany him so, despite his state of shock, he made the journey alone. I guess the following two hours on the train and London underground were two of the longest hours of his life.

I was not aware of that first visit, nor his subsequent daily visits, as I was in an induced coma. A couple of weeks later, I regained consciousness in the intensive care unit of the Royal London Hospital. I had no idea why I was there, how I got there or how long I had been there. I felt very comfortable and had no pain; I think it seemed dark but I felt no panic or worry about my situation. Colin was there with me; in fact, he was the only visitor I was allowed. I couldn't understand why, I didn't feel ill so I couldn't be that bad. Whatever had happened?

Obviously I had been in some kind of serious accident. I shudder now to imagine how Colin felt when he first set eyes on me in hospital. My scull and right side of my head and face were so severely damaged I would not have been surprised if he thought it would mean the end of our life together as we knew it. It must have been hard to believe that I could escape brain damage with those injuries.

I had absolutely no idea what had happened to me and I don't even remember asking but I had survived whatever it was. Somehow Colin found the courage to tell me that I had lost my left arm above the elbow and slowly I learned about my numerous injuries. I had lost most of my scalp, and skin from both my thighs was grafted onto my head. My right eye was badly damaged and my right ear had gone. I had a very long scar on my knee and more skin grafting under my left armpit and my right little finger had been grafted back onto my hand. What a mess. Despite all this I felt very positive and safe and above all I had no pain and, seemingly, nothing to worry about. When I was told I had been admitted with multiple injuries, believe it or not, I found this slightly amusing, like something you read in the newspaper – it couldn't be me.

The truth was that I had been airlifted to the Royal London Hospital after a fall onto the train tracks at my local station which left me barely breathing, with irreparable damage to my right eye and ear, severe electrical burns to my body, multiple broken bones and life threatening bleeding.

On arrival in A&E I was aggressively fluid resuscitated, before being rushed into emergency surgery that lasted many hours. In theatre, surgeons had to make the heart-breaking decision to amputate my left arm in order to save my life. I fell into a coma and it was at least two weeks before I woke up.

One of my early recollections is of a nurse standing by my bed with a plastic box in one hand and a pair of tweezers in the other. I was positioned with my head raised and as I lay there she was repeatedly picking something out of the box and carefully placing it on my head. At one point I was aware of something falling from my head and landing with a plop on my chest; it was a leech. How incredible, my head wounds were being treated with leeches, a healing therapy that can be traced back to the second century BC!

I also remember the stitches being taken out of the wound on my left knee, it was a right angled gash about seven inches long – a real shark attack scar. The first time I saw my "little arm" it was healed. I wondered just however long had I been in hospital.

My jigsaw puzzle of injuries meant I had to be treated by specialist teams from across the capital including plastic and maxillofacial surgeons from The Royal London and St Bartholomew's Hospital. My most difficult injuries to treat were the high voltage burns to my head, face and jaw, which had left me virtually unrecognizable. My head was so severely damaged that plastic surgeons had to rebuild part of my skull. Professor of Academic Plastic Surgery Simon Myers, who carried out the procedure, explained that when he first saw me, the right side of my skull had been severely damaged by the high voltage current that had entered my left arm, damaging it irreparably, crossed my heart, and then exited through my right temple causing dramatic soft tissue damage. In fact the bone was burnt almost to the level of the brain and at the time of my rescue the fluid was bubbling. A moment longer and methinks my brains would have been boiled.

I'm sure it won't come as a surprise to know that I have since read a bit about such burns. I have learned that between the entrance and exit points of an electric current hidden destruction of deeper tissues can occur. An electric current can injure almost every organ system of the body. Such electrically conductive burns are simply thermal injuries occurring when the electric energy is converted to thermal energy. A moment longer and methinks my internal organs would have been fried.

All the dead skin was cut away to carefully uncover the delicate, very thin layer of skull bone beneath. My skull was then covered with synthetic skin, and my unburned scalp was moved around to get the area to heal. Skin was borrowed from my thighs to close the secondary wounds. Maxillofacial trauma surgeon Mr Simon Holmes painstakingly sculpted a new cheekbone and eyebrow for me. In describing this challenging process he said the whole side of my head was damaged, including the large muscle that facilitated opening and closing my mouth. The electric current that had passed through this muscle had turned it into a stiff leather-like band, which prevented me from opening my mouth. This had to be removed along with part of the dead cheekbone and lower jaw.

I still had round-the-clock care when I was moved to the high dependency unit where my journey of recovery really began. The multi-disciplinary team involved in my care included a trauma team of vascular and orthopaedic surgeons, plastic surgeons, maxillofacial surgeons, neurology surgeons, ophthalmologist, orthoptist, ear nose and throat surgeons, nurse specialist in burns and plastic surgery, physiotherapists, occupational therapists and a psychologist.

I shared the ward with three other patients and although nursing care was on hand twenty-four seven, Colin was concerned enough to have a word with the Sister in charge about the company I was keeping. I don't recall being at all fazed by this but I could understand Colin's concern.

One of the patients opposite me was not a happy bunny. Although he had both legs in plaster he still managed to get himself out of bed and try to escape in a wheelchair. Just as well he didn't speak English very clearly; he wasn't in a mood to be polite. The other patient opposite me was a victim of street crime and had been shot. He was okay and when his noisy Caribbean family visitors arrived at visiting times it was quite an occasion. They were very friendly and one lady wore lovely bright scarves on her head, which I admired. One day she presented me with a couple of scarves she no longer wanted. How kind and thoughtful was that? I was obviously going to need a means of covering my head one day.

The patient in the bed adjacent to me was a victim of aggravated burglary and he had apparently been 'done over' with a Stanley knife. I gleaned all this information from the conversations he had with the two policemen who were visiting him. However, the patient didn't seem interested in the police; he just kept asking for the photographer to record the evidence of his injuries.

Undoubtedly drug induced but I slept a great deal during the next few weeks. It felt like a wonderful, deep, healing sleep. The efficient professionalism of the staff left no room for embarrassment, although

I will never forget Colin's face when he realised the tall Nigerian male nurse he had seen in the ward had washed his wife that morning! It wasn't long before he felt as I did – so grateful that I was being so well looked after by such compassionate, wonderful people. I felt my recovery was being nurtured and therefore it endorsed my belief that my life was worthy of saving. I must have sometimes awoken in the night because I remember a Filipino nurse sitting by my bedside and when we looked at each other he quietly said "Divine intervention". Do I believe in it? It's a very personal question but I know how I feel now when I think about my life, how I am loved and what I survived. My existence was preserved and I have the knowledge, through experience, that life can be worth living again after a major crisis.

I was introduced to the surgeon who told me he had to make a life-changing decision for both of us when he had to amputate my arm. I felt sympathy for him – imagine having to make decisions like that in your daily work – but the saddest fact for me was that I could no longer wear my wedding ring. Although that still saddens me, I would love to meet that surgeon again to be able to tell him I'm okay and how my life-changing experience has now actually enriched my life.

The dressing on my right eye was changed every four hours then every eight hours for several weeks but sadly, unlike me, it did not survive and I gave my consent for its removal. Even this did not send me into a panic, I seemed to be coping ok with one eye, but I'll admit to being emotional after the operation – the loss of an eye is quite profound, not only for seeing properly but also for affecting what I looked like.

Some of my clinic appointments were at St Bartholomew's Hospital and I was transported by ambulance or taxi with an escort nurse accompanying me. I thought this was great, it was an outing and reminded me of how much I had enjoyed coach trips when I was a child. It also reminded me that life was still going on out there, the

London streets were buzzing with people and traffic. Several times I had the same taxi driver and he would point out places of interest en route. We passed the Whitechapel Bell Foundry, the old church of St Bartholomew the Great and, via a little detour for my benefit, we even crossed Tower Bridge one day.

After my appointments I would have to wait in the hospital patient transport area for my transport back to The Royal London. On one occasion the receptionist suggested I could wait in another room away from the other sick and injured patients. Whatever her motive was, I appreciated the gesture and accepted her offer of privacy. On my return, I related this to a fellow patient and was surprised by her reaction. She was horrified that the receptionist had seen fit to suggest a private room for me so that the sight of me wouldn't upset the other patients! What an example of how the same scenario can be interpreted so differently.

When not being pushed on a bed to the operating theatre I was pushed in a wheelchair to various clinic appointments within the Royal London, such was my mode of hospital transport. My reflection in a glass framed picture in one of the corridors gave me my first hint of my appearance. The elaborate dressing encasing my head was reminiscent of a frill round a birthday or Christmas cake.

My scalp was proving the most difficult to heal and I was given two choices: Have an operation to remove a muscle from my back and place it over my wound, or have a vac-pump attached to my head for a couple of weeks. I chose the latter and under general anaesthetic a membrane skullcap was fitted to my head. It had a tube leading to a pump where all the muck and debris from my wound was sucked off, thus encouraging the blood supply to promote healing; the modern version of leeches, I guess. When my daughter saw me she suggested I could be an extra on Dr Who. What a cheek, but also what a relief that humour was beginning to return to our lives.

The main problem was that the vac-pump was a fairly weighty piece of equipment, which plugged into the mains. This meant I could not move far from my bed or go to the loo unless a nurse carried it around for me. It was one of the youngest nurses in the ward who had the bright idea of strapping my machine to a drip stand. Wonderful, for short trips, I could now pull the plug from the wall, hold the flex and wheel my vac-pump around with me while it worked on its own battery. What a difference this made. All was well until one visiting time when Colin kept giving me funny looks; he didn't want to worry me but said my head appeared to be a different shape. There seemed to be a big depression on one side and it was higher in the front. We tried not to panic or cause alarm, it did not give me any discomfort but what could be the reason for my head appearing to contort itself? We decided we had to call a nurse to come and investigate. Apparently my pump had not been plugged back in after one of my trips to the bathroom and my dressing was deflating.

Each dressing change, usually twice a week, meant a trip to the operating theatre. I didn't know this when I chose the vac-pump! The sunny side of this though was when I told the anaesthetist we should stop meeting like this. He took my hand, leaned over and looked me in the eye and said, "people will say we're in love". I love that moment and there were many such moments of verbal banter that provided me with a wonderful feeling of not only being alive but more importantly, being part of life. Life is nothing without feeling; I felt acutely aware that the good feelings I now experienced were a great contrast to how I felt before this happened to me. I could remember when I felt like I was living in a cocoon, in agony and unable to function properly or feel any emotion. My personal worries had spiralled overwhelmingly out of proportion, robbing me of any pleasure and turning my life into a living hell.

Obviously I was 'nil by mouth' on the day of my dressing change operation and on more than one occasion my operation had to be rescheduled for another day. Whilst this played havoc with my diet and my sugar level it was understandable; mine was hardly a case of life or death. Whenever I heard the air ambulance helicopter approaching the hospital I guessed my operation might be cancelled for that day and I wondered how many operations I had disrupted the day I had been an emergency patient on board the approaching helicopter.

The vac-pump was finally removed after seven weeks. It had done its job and my scalp was healing at last. I asked why the tight brown plastic was left on my head and the nurses looked at me quizzically – it was my head! I didn't know what new grafted skin looked like and didn't know what to expect. Seeing myself in a mirror for the first time brought my first real tears. In the dark days before my accident I had been unable to cry and I had not really cried until now and it felt good, like the start of my feelings coming back.

Regrettably, my right hand little finger was not looking very healthy. In fact, it was not doing well at all so it had to be amputated. I returned from the operating theatre plastered from my fingertips to my elbow, thus rendered completely helpless. Until this point my main sustenance had been administered via a tube up my nose. What joy when the doctor said he could remove the tube providing I had at least four vitamin milk drinks a day – no problem; unlike most of the patients, I actually liked them, especially the cappuccino flavour and I could certainly suck through a straw. However, I had a very nasty shock when a nurse tried to spoon-feed me. I was horrified to discover that it was impossible to open my mouth any wider than it was necessary to speak. I now even had to be fed and this was not easy as injury to my jaw and surrounding muscles had seriously compromised my ability to open my mouth. Being spoon-fed, I might add, demanded a large amount of tolerance on my part. I suggested that anyone feeding a patient ought themselves to be spoon-fed. Food seemed to be coming at me at different levels and at different speeds. Not being able to feed myself was a big frustration.

I was given some wooden lollypop sticks like the ones doctors use to depress your tongue when they want to see down your throat. I had to force them between my teeth and with great difficulty another stick was added every day. Later I was presented with a gadget called a Therabite to force my mouth open for as long and as often as I could bear it. A long period of self-physiotherapy eventually helped me regain the movement so I could eat and speak as normal. It really was self-inflicted torture and progress was frustratingly slow. The therabite came home with me when I left hospital and I had to continue this torture for several months before I felt real movement. What an amazing moment that was; I was getting somewhere at last. I was still living on pureed food and custard but I was beginning to push soft food like cake and bread into my mouth. As I reported to the surgeons at my appointments after my discharge, I could eat for survival but not socially. It was about fifteen months after I left hospital that my eating was socially acceptable. I can still remember where and when I ate my first sandwich. I was in a café in Frinton on Sea in Essex where we had gone to see a memorial seat, overlooking the sea, erected in memory of Colin's parents who had passed away a few years earlier. They had run a modern sequence dance club in the area for many years.

It was also at this time that I experienced pain for the first time since I had been admitted to hospital. Interestingly enough it was nothing to do with my injuries. It became excruciating painful to go to the loo. With both my arms out of action I had to wait in agony for a nurse to assist me in using a commode. I remember one night screaming in pain; it was not a pain I could keep to myself. At this point I must tell you about the commode that collapsed one night. The only good thing about it was that the 'pot' fell right through to the floor before my performance started. Thank goodness!

It seemed that the reason for my severe discomfort was a urine infection. Before this was confirmed, however, I was moved to an isolation room and had to have a colonoscopy. What an experience that was. I wasn't looking forward to it but I found it fascinating seeing inside my tubes. I watched the entire procedure on a screen, like being on the telly but not as we know it. A polyp was seen along the way and promptly zapped away on the return. When I related this experience to a nurse she said I must be the only patient ever to be excited about having had a colonoscopy.

My move to a general ward heralded a new chapter in my slow return to normality. My temporary home for the next few months was Treves Ward. Treves was the name of the surgeon in the 1880s who had the famous Joseph Merrick, known as the elephant man, in his care. This irony was not lost on me and the fact that I could relate to disfigurement with a hint of sardonic humour gave me assurance that my mind was recovering as well as my body.

At last I was gaining some independence and had regular visits from occupational therapists and physiotherapists. I started to feed myself and eventually wash myself but always with a nurse escort when I had a shower – the risk of a fall was quite high. While having a shower one day I felt a wave of emotion come over me and I started to cry. Tears flowed freely and the nurse asked if I wanted to talk to someone. "Oh yes please, yes I do." My words fell eagerly out of my mouth and I felt great relief that I was being offered the opportunity to unburden myself; at last salvation was on the way. I had been in hospital for a couple of months and was fully aware of my situation and yet almost felt like I was in a dream. This could have been because of my medication but I remember feeling at that time like I was slowly thawing out while feelings and emotions were gradually returning.

Soon after my tearful episode in the shower I started to have regular visits from a psychiatrist and it was a great comfort to have a professional confidante, independent of my family and friends. I learned that I was rescued from a railway line by the air ambulance and flown by helicopter to the Royal London Hospital. I could not believe it, I had no memory whatsoever of leaving home that morning, of where I was going or what I was wearing. I asked Colin what was missing from my wardrobe!

Poor Colin. I was only just beginning to realise what he and the rest of my family was going through. Before the accident I just could not tell Colin how I felt. I just thought that if I was not there he would not have to worry about me anymore. But now I could tell the psychiatrist how terrified I had been of the world news and modern technology, I could tell him everything about my illness that I had not been able to talk about before. I knew he would not judge me or try to control me. How valuable to have someone like that to confide in. It seems a strange contradiction that I could tell a stranger my innermost thoughts and yet had been unable to confide in my nearest and dearest. Had I been able to confide I may have spared them all the horrors of my accident and all the anguish that went with the weeks during which my survival was in doubt. In my efforts to spare family and friends their worry I seemed to have managed to increase the intensity of it. This anomaly occupied my thoughts a lot but as I improved physically and emotionally I hoped that I would be forgiven and accepted after what had happened to me.

I was of an age to remember that what I had apparently attempted was once a criminal offence and I was allowing myself to feel a degree of shame and embarrassment. Whilst I didn't really believe this was justified, I almost felt as though I deserved to be punished. Something had happened to me that threatened my very existence and changed my life forever and yet I could not recall any of it.

I carried this burden with me in the very back of my mind. How could I freely enjoy the wonderful life I was discovering on the other side of hell? Did I have to pay a penalty for what I had done? I tried to mitigate my actions, telling myself I had been ill, my life was distorted, it was corrupt and surely it wasn't my fault. Something had happened to unbalance my perspective of life to make it scary, ugly and unwanted.

While I was in hospital I indulged in one of my favourite occupations, lying in bed whilst listening to Radio 4. I listened intently when I heard an episode of Woman's Hour featuring depression. Why did this illness, which affected such a large percentage of the population, have such a stigma? It should be given a higher profile and discussed more openly if there is ever going to be a deeper understanding of helping sufferers. A quick remedy for feeling down or having an attack of the grumps can be to have a treat or indulgence. In the long run this is only a short-term solution and the low mood inevitably returns. In my experience severe depression only has one answer and that is a permanent solution, one that will end such suffering forever. I know that's what I wanted because my suffering was so intense it seemed the only guaranteed way out. I don't think I could have been convinced that there was another way and that I could ever feel well again. The severity of my infirmity seemed only to heighten my fear and distress of the consequences of being mentally ill. It could mean committal to a mental hospital. Although the days of mental asylums were past the knowledge of them could still haunt my generation. At school in the 1950s children would chant and tease each other about the 'nut house'. I am finding it hard to write these words, I don't really want to commit them to paper, yet feel I must tell all truthfully.

Physical and emotional support in hospital was brilliant, the Royal London staff were there for me every step of the way. I felt their timing of introducing each step of my recovery was just right.

I was quite surprised by my emotional reaction when taken to the kitchen area to try out some basic catering skills. It seemed so long since I had seen a kitchen sink, not to mention a cooker or a kettle. I succeeded in making a cup of coffee and a jam sandwich for myself without too much difficulty but failed to peel a potato, the poor vegetable was impaled on a spiked board and massacred by my attempts to skin it alive with a potato peeler. Not that it bothered me because one of my favourite foods is a jacket potato.

I was given a small plastic tub containing something similar to play dough. It was bright yellow and I had to squeeze it in my hand to exercise my fingers. Adjusting to the one eye and one arm way of doing things was quite a challenge. Although I gained the strength to lift my full water jug I couldn't be trusted to pour the water into the mug. I discovered this to my cost when I actually poured water all over the table across my bed, consequently and uncomfortably, wetting my bedding! The exact location of a vessel takes time to judge correctly when you only have one eye. Similarly, cutting with scissors or accepting something being given to me could leave me snipping or grasping at thin air! I also had to learn to write again, and I had various surfaces from soft velvet to sandpaper with which to de-sensitise my little finger wound.

My first attempt to walk was really frightening. Why wouldn't my legs support my body anymore and why wouldn't they move in the direction I wanted them to? A doctor with a hammer checked my reflexes and said it was only muscle wastage. I found it hard to believe him but given time and lots of physiotherapy and exercise, he was proved right. I was quite excited when presented with a cycling machine and I was able to sit on the edge of my bed and pedal for ten minutes solid at least once a day.

Before I was allowed to tackle walking up and down stairs, I was given an obstacle course of items such as a bucket, a chair and a jug, etc to walk around without bumping into anything and then pick up things from the floor without falling over.

I felt envious of a lady in the ward who was over ninety years old, who would return from the gym saying she had muscles like Pop-eye. It wasn't only her muscles I was jealous of it was the fact that she was going to the gym. Eventually I was deemed ready and it was my turn at last. Two lovely young physiotherapists stood at the foot of my bed one day and said they could take me to the gym. They had eyes as bright as buttons and smiles to match and I couldn't wait to start my exercise regime.

My favourite piece of equipment, of course, was the bike. I was thrilled to be doing something familiar that I loved. Without leaving the room I was cycling and even going uphill. I also had a go at hitting balls with a tennis racquet – it was fun even if it was a bit hit and miss! My most vivid memory of being in the gym is when I was told to lie on the floor. To my great satisfaction I was able to do this and felt quite pleased with myself. Then I was told to get up, by myself, without any help. Needless to say, I struggled, and struggled, and struggled. My physiotherapist sat watching me and did nothing to help me, other than verbal encouragement. She called it tough love and when I eventually got myself on my feet, exhausted and gasping, I had learned that tough love worked and it was the best kind of love for self-esteem.

Another physiotherapist explained mirror box therapy to me in regard to my amputated arm and asked if I would like to try it. I was intrigued and of course I was willing to try it. She brought me a wooden box with a mirror fixed to one side. The box was placed on a table, I sat at the table and placed my little arm in the box, positioned so that I could see the reflection of my right arm and hand in the mirror. The exercise was to move my right hand and fingers, watch the reflection and visualize the same movement happening in my amputated left hand. I was fascinated with this therapy and soon found that totally focusing on making my left hand and fingers 'move' seemed very positive and beneficial. Sometimes some of my 'invisible fingers' were reasonably flexible but at other times my hand would feel frozen and it wasn't even possible to open my fingers. One of these mirror box sessions took place in the gym and on this occasion the physiotherapist said she would let me carry on with the exercises on my own for a couple of minutes. When she returned she really made me jump in surprise, I was so engrossed I was totally unaware of her return after about ten minutes as she had not wanted to interrupt my concentration. I soon realised I could close my eye and visualise my hand exercises without using the mirror box and frequently did so before going to sleep.

I was taking medication to alleviate any phantom pain from my missing arm. The main feeling I had, however, was a strong sensation rather like a bad attack of nettle stings which really only bothered me when I talked or thought about it. Mainly my non-existent arm felt sort of numb and my hand felt like it was at about elbow height. That is not to say that I never experienced any phantom pain. Fortunately it was not very often but when it happened it was excruciating and to make it worse there was nothing I could touch or hold for comfort. Imagine an electric shock being administered to your left hand while your right hand is tied behind your back – it really is akin to torture.

My five months in hospital were very rewarding, giving me an insight into human nature I would otherwise never have experienced. Some fellow patients were inspirational and some were in need of inspiration. People watching is always a fascinating pastime, none more so than in hospital. I had a front row seat while all the characters played their cameo roles before me: the larger than life black lady who had a different hairstyle every day as she worked her way through her wardrobe of wigs but refused to talk to her anxious daughter on the hospital phone. "What's the point, I don't know when I'm going home" was her response to the poor nurse relaying messages; the patient whose husband disappeared behind his newspaper during visits while she talked loudly to other patients and then he fell asleep on her bed while they waited for her medication the day she was discharged; the young lady worried about her pet dog while her partner was in charge of their house move; Kelly, the petite, young, victim of a cycle accident who occupied the bed opposite me and amazed me with her trips out of the hospital with her friends. How I envied Kelly the plates of fresh salad she devoured when I was unable to eat properly. When she was due to be discharged from hospital I knew I would miss her. I didn't even get to say goodbye as I was fast asleep when she left. However, the chair by my bed was laden with goodies from her, including magazines, hand cream, cooling spray and her lovely china mug that I had admired.

I need not have worried – before too long Kelly was back as an inpatient again and so began a friendship that endures to this day.

Being unwell or injured in unfamiliar surroundings and with strangers for company is enough to sap anyone's confidence. New patients were understandably nervous and often uncooperative especially if there was a language difference. It was interesting to note how much more relaxed people were by their third or fourth day, by which time conversations had been struck up with fellow patients and they were more familiar with the hospital routine.

My sympathy went out to the nursing staff, who plainly did not have enough time to tend to all needs at all times. One thing I learned as a patient is to have patience. Hospital care cannot always be one to one.

I consider myself one of the luckiest patients, not only for surviving, but also for all the friends who made the long journey to London see me, and my husband, Colin, who came every single day for five months. I really enjoyed visiting time and appreciated the distance friends had come and the time they were spending on coming to see me. Sometimes it almost felt like I was having a party with Colin and a couple of friends round my bed all laughing and joking. "Don't know what you're on, Lin, but we'd love some" was often said.

When September came round my birthday was imminent but there was no sign of me going home yet. So it was that my sixty-third birthday was spent in hospital and Colin and my daughter both visited me. When my daughter went off to the toilet I reassured Colin that it didn't bother me to be in hospital for my birthday, but he suggested we might have a proper celebration the following year anyway. Suddenly bells started ringing very loudly – had Colin organized a surprise strip-a-gram or was it a fire alarm? Alas, it was the latter and apprehension started to spread in the ward.

What does one grab first if one has to evacuate the building, I wondered, but my concern didn't seem to match what was going on before my eyes. Kelly and my daughter were entering the ward with a hospital trolley laden with party food including a cake ablaze with birthday candles. Completely without my knowledge this impromptu party had been arranged with full consent of the Ward Sister, but unfortunately their planning had not taken into account the possibility of smoke from the candles setting off the fire alarms. It turned out to be one of my best, never to be forgotten, birthday surprises ever.

It was quite an event the first time Colin took me to the coffee shop on the ground floor of the hospital. I may not have looked amazing with one arm and my head extensively bandaged but I can assure you, I actually felt amazing. I was having a coffee with Colin when not so long ago I was scared to drink it. How normally brilliant was that? It seemed even more amazing when Colin and I left the hospital building one day with two friends who were visiting me and we all went to a café down the road. Still bandaged up, but I was actually carefully walking down the road, mingling with the public. It was an exciting achievement for me as we took our seats in a café and ordered coffee. I remember my friend had a piece of chocolate cake but I did not as I still couldn't eat politely at that time.

Before my illness started we had booked seats for a Cliff Richard concert at Wembley, celebrating his fifty years in show business. No need to be sorry, we thought, it's not until November, I'll be home by then. Weeks were passing, however, and by the end of October there was still no prospect of a discharge date. We considered finding someone else to have our tickets but held onto the hope that we would be able to go to the concert.

Yes, I did go to the concert, the nurses were my fairy godmothers and helped to dress me and tied my best scarf elegantly round my head. My golden carriage was a taxi and my Prince Charming was Colin. He had arranged everything down to the last detail. I was warned to take extra care particularly on stairs and not get upset if people stared at me or even made comments. Nobody did and to be honest I was so caught up in my own world of excitement I wouldn't have been upset if they had done.

I shudder to think how much the whole adventure cost with a taxi to and from the hospital to Wembley Stadium but we agreed it was worth every penny. Cliff did not disappoint, it was a wonderful show and I felt like a real life Cinderella creeping back to my humble abode just before midnight after my night out at the palace!

While I was in hospital I received more than a hundred cards and letters from friends and learned that prayers were being said for me in our local church and in Lincolnshire Cathedral. This outpouring of love and support for me was overwhelming. During her visit one day my good friend and neighbour Donna told me of a lady she had met crying in the church. On asking if she was all right the lady said she was crying for a friend who had had an accident and was in hospital. Although they did not know each other I knew them both. It was another dear friend Margaret and yes, I was that friend in hospital. It was wonderful when Donna brought her two young daughters, Shannon and Eliza, to see me one day. It wasn't long before my discharge and when I said they were not to worry if I looked a bit different when I came home, Eliza, who was about seven at the time, made my day by quickly saying "But you'll still be the same ol' Lin". My only concern was for all the anxiety I had caused, I had no worries then or now about how I would cope with my disabilities – I had survived and life felt good.

It's never a good time to have an accident but I was grateful that this had not happened to me earlier in my life. It was a huge relief to be retired, I didn't have to worry about time off work or having to face work colleagues on my return, nor possibly having to look for another job. I also felt grateful that both my parents and Colin's parents were no longer alive. I would hate to have caused them grief.

I couldn't help thinking that if my accident had not happened I would still have all the bits and pieces I was born with but I doubt that I would have the appreciation of life that I currently felt. I may have lost a few physical parts but I recall responding to a fellow hospital patient's sympathetic concern by saying "But I've got my life back". I can now feel emotion, gone is the anxiety, the fear and blackness; I am alive and one hundred per cent happy about it.

It would seem an obvious thought that my depression could return and obviously it is a thought that has occurred to me. That thought does not worry me, however. If anything I believe I am less likely to suffer the same again than someone who has never had depression. For those who have not experienced depression I feel it is too scary to understand or believe what is happening. I now know the signs and can tell the difference between a disappointment, a frustration or a mood that I will eventually get over and something that is really not right and out of proportion for more a day or two. In my experience it developed so slowly and felt such a strange encounter that I challenged my own belief in what was happening because it was too frightening. I feel so much stronger now knowing I have contacts I can call upon and my first point of call, without hesitation, would be a professional such as my psychiatric doctor or counsellor. I know I would not again allow myself a period of denial, thinking I would get better on my own.

It is said you only live once and that life is a gift and the only certainty in life is death. But I feel I have been twice blessed with the gift of life and I keenly needed to say thank you. Mistakenly believing that my rescuers were the London Air Ambulance we made a donation to them and I got their T-shirt in the hospital shop. I also asked if it would be possible to meet the crew who had saved me. In fact it had been the Kent Surrey and Sussex Air Ambulance who flew to my rescue (another donation and another T-shirt) but incredibly the doctor who attended me had since transferred to the Royal London Hospital so it was possible that I could meet him.

Seated on the bed of fellow patient Kelly one day and having a good old chat when I heard my name called – "Linda, I have a visitor for you" – I turned round to see a tall, dark, handsome stranger entering the ward with the Ward Sister. I heard someone say "Oh my god! He's drop dead gorgeous!" and instantly realised the words had come out of my own mouth. How embarrassing was that?

So it was that I was introduced to the doctor who had saved my life, although he insisted quite rightly that he was one of a team. It was wonderful to be able to say thank you and express how grateful I was. He explained that it was wonderful to hear my words because often they have to work without the patient's permission and sometimes against the patient's will.

I am almost at a loss to put into words exactly how I felt at meeting this man. With his team, in very difficult circumstances, he had the knowledge, skill and ability to know exactly what to do, when to do it and how to do it in order to preserve my existence and get me to the right hospital in time to save my life. How lucky was I to be delivered into the capable, caring hands of the amazing trauma team at the Royal London Hospital. I remember absolutely nothing of that fateful event but will be eternally grateful for my eventual good fortune on that day.

I have no true explanation of what happened and still find it hard to believe. I obviously thought about it and considered various scenarios and wondered exactly how it happened. I declined the opportunity of seeing CCTV footage, though, knowing that would give me an image in my mind. No way would I take the risk of suffering flashbacks to haunt me. I did learn another amazing fact, however, when Colin told me a railway ticket was among my personal items returned to him. The ticket was a standard cheap day return from Godalming to Portsmouth costing ten pounds and valid for one day only: 7 July 2008. I obviously wanted to come back.

CHAPTER XII

Out of hospital

My discharge date from The Royal London Hospital was 11 November 2008, after five months as an inpatient. My discharge form was full of information about my injuries; the main condition treated was stated as severe electrical burns to face, scalp and left arm. It also listed my ongoing medication; I had seven different drugs to make up my future daily cocktail.

I had missed the summer at home and autumn was in full swing, but it was good to be home with all my familiar home comforts. Everything was still there and Colin had done a sterling job of looking after our home in my absence. He had worked out and kept to a great routine of shopping and housework and keeping up with the laundry, etc and packing a sandwich lunch for himself to eat on the train every day. Much as he was relieved to have me back home and not have to travel to London every day, his worry was not completely over; I imagine I must have been quite a responsibility for him.

Once again I could see the beautiful view from our bedroom window, which also meant I could see the railway line. Would it evoke memories of my past and remind me how I felt the last time I saw it? Thankfully it did not. My spirit felt uplifted, what joy to survive and find my life before my illness was still there, not only materially but emotionally too.

Although I was no longer an inpatient I still needed medical attention after I came home. The District Nurse called every day for a couple of weeks to change the dressings on my head wound that was far from fully healed. Gradually this responsibility was transferred to Colin who rose to the challenge admirably as always. The skin grafting donor sites on my thighs still had to be generously creamed twice a day so it was easier to wrap a bath towel around me than to wear trousers. After several weeks of feeling like the proverbial woman in a dressing gown I was able to start thinking about dressing properly to start going out. This was still quite challenging but I found it easier to cope with the outside world while I was still an obvious patient with my head swathed in bandages. When they were no longer necessary it became trickier. How do I face the world now without looking odd?

Despite feeling like a hint of an incognito Hollywood star, scarves and dark glasses were my best confidence boosters when going out. I had been given some scarves while I was in hospital and now, with every appointment there, I was discovering the huge choice of very inexpensive, lovely scarves available on the Asian market stalls opposite the Royal London Hospital. An alternative solution was to wear a Buff on my head. This was a tube of stretchy stockinette fabric, which could be worn in a variety of ways. I had at least ten of them in various colours and patterns and wore them like a skull-cap, pulled down to cover my right eye socket. I did decide that my black and white striped T-shirt had to go when I realised that I was looking a bit like a pirate.

I was fully aware of my culinary limitations so I avoided the kitchen. Fortunately Colin was happy to prepare our meals, so I did my best not to interfere. Even though I was now home, I still felt like a patient and Colin was wonderful at looking after me. The full impact of my arm amputation didn't seem to have sunk in as I was still having so much done for me. Nevertheless, in my head I felt that if I couldn't do something I wanted to do, in time I knew I would find a way.

Making a mistake is often heralded as the best way to learn; by experience. I can honestly say I have certainly learned a lot from my experience. Never again will I keep negative thoughts to myself. I recognise my depression as a real illness and, of course, cannot rule out not being ill again but I know the warning signs now and believe that I would try everything possible to never ever allow myself to sink into those depths of despair again. I have learned the true value of life and do not take any of it for granted. It is just like the end of the children's nursery rhyme; when it's good, it's very, very good and when it's bad it's horrid. Far from thinking it is weak to admit that you need help, I see it as a sign of strength and wisdom to seek help and seek it sooner rather than later. Much wiser than exhausting yourself until there is no power left in your battery.

If your petrol is running low, top up at the FIRST garage you encounter. You may not find one when your fuel level is critical.

I came across a piece of paper bearing the following three lines, apparently I wrote them during my depression but do not remember doing so. I must have had a lucid moment in my despair, because I feel they summed up my feelings perfectly:

- The past is too perfect
- The present is too painful
- The future is too frightening

If you can overcome your demons and survive you can help others and earn yourself the freedom to have a more richly rewarding life than you could ever possibly imagine. A rich, rewarding life is exactly what I have got. It's fascinating to discover how to adapt and cope with challenges.

I acknowledge the power of confidence and self-esteem. It virtually controls my life and is fundamental to my wellbeing, it has the power to reward and I know how it feels to be rewarded. Total loss of confidence for me meant being robbed of the joy of life. I know how it feels to be robbed.

Confidence is uniquely precious, don't lose it nurture it, talk to it and it will grow. Body language speaks louder than words and tells the truth. Be posture aware, stand tall, shoulders back and look the world in the eye. Life is not a competition; we are all different so why waste energy trying to be like someone else? Use all of yours to promote your best wellbeing. Highlighting one's best feature is better than focusing on imperfections.

Confidence can be convincingly faked and why not? Accept a challenge then work out how to deal with it then reward yourself for your achievement. Result: confidence to accept another challenge. I have accepted challenges and felt the fulfilment of success. I won't give up at any setbacks. Tenacity is the name of the game.

Be generous, help others and be rewarded by seeing their confidence grow. I believe in giving back to those who helped me.

Whenever I think about my life now I get a feeling inside that I call my soda fountain effect. It fills me with happiness and elation. I have the confidence to say no without having to justify my decision. With confidence there is no such thing as negativity.

Be	Committed	honest and loyal to yourself always. Stand by your opinions and have the confidence/power to change them if you want to.
Be	Objective	focus on your target
Not be	Negative	
Be	Fantastic	feel fantastic because you are
Be	Inquisitive	discover your own answers. Don't be inhibited – ASK!
Be	Delightful	relish the delight of living
Be	Emotional	Savour your spectrum of feelings
Not be	Negative	
Be	Caring	give more receive more
Be	Ego	be yourself

There are two points of view to even the worst experience. I am aware and mindful but living in fear that something bad might happen is allowing fear to steal my joy. I would become both offender and victim and my fears may be unfounded. When faced with a problem these days I ask myself what is the worst-case scenario of my situation? If my fears were founded it would be a terrible experience but my fear would then be replaced by my coping mechanism and positive thinking.

I was thrilled to discover I could use my beloved sewing machine and when we moved house, promptly ordered fabric for new curtains. "Who's going to make them?" my husband asked. "I am," I replied, and I did, plus making a fitted seat cushion for a bench, painting and re-upholstering a Lloyd Loom bedroom chair and laundry basket and, as I had some fabric left over, I made a bag for my hairdryer, just for good measure!

I could hardly believe it when a friend asked if I could make her some new cushions. She had not only requested new cushions, she had paid me a huge compliment by trusting my ability and I doubt that she could have realised what a boost this was for my confidence. Likewise, when a friend asked if I could make a small alteration to her daughter's dress for her college ball. It was such a delight to carry out this task and a real thrill to be so trusted.

I had discovered that by using my sewing machine on the floor with the foot pedal under my right leg, I freed my right hand to guide the material and my left leg became my left 'arm'. Fortunately I have always been very flexible and found this modus operandi quite comfortable. In fact, several times I was so wrapped up in my sewing that my left foot actually felt like I was using my left hand.

At one of my many outpatient appointments at the RLH and St Bartholomew's Hospitals it was suggested I might tell my story. I must say this idea appealed to me and I felt more than happy to celebrate my survival from a medical point of view as well as my new-found joy of life. In collaboration with two consultants, I worked on some text for a press release, emailing our words back and forward to each other for editing and approval. I was still wondering which newspaper would carry my story when I had a phone call from the hospital press office one Monday morning; saying they had decided to pitch it at TV instead. What a surprise, and three days later Colin and I were being interviewed in our own home. When they wanted to film me doing something in the home, I agreed as long as it wasn't just stirring a mug of coffee in the kitchen. The cameraman started to clear space on the table when I suggested using my sewing machine. He soon realised his mistake when I set up my machine on the floor.

The Channel 5 news crew left soon after midday saying that my story would be featured on their evening news that day, providing there were no ground-breaking events to knock me out of their headlines. Well, the queen did not abdicate and the sky did not fall in so I did hit the headlines.

The newsreader introduced me as a woman who had survived some of the worst injuries that the trauma team had ever seen. I don't believe that, I thought, she's exaggerating for the sake of effect. However, after watching the surgeon's input and seeing the X-ray showing the damage to my scull, I began to believe there might be some truth in the announcer's statement. Of course, I believed I had suffered serious injuries but I had felt so good all the time ever since, I just could not relate to the seriousness of it all. Only now did I begin to understand what all the fuss was about – my survival and recovery really did seem like a miracle.

Everything I experience now is wonderful – whether I see it, smell it or hear it, there seems to be almost a novelty affect. It is all so exciting that I lead a virtually normal life despite my disability and I can appreciate and feel it emotionally. I admit that I have never mastered the art of vegetable peeling but I am so lucky to have a husband who prepares all our meals. I can cope with changing the sheets on the bed, still doing 'hospital corners', and enjoy doing the ironing as I always have done. I confess to breaking a few ornaments while trying to dust them but that just means there are fewer things to dust.

I will always try to be independent but obviously there are times when Colin is not with me and help is necessary. I have yet to find a stranger who is not willing to help, whether it is holding something for me or doing up my trouser button in a public loo. Sometimes people go into 'parent mode' and assistance feels like it is verging on patronising but I try to accept it graciously. I don't think remarks like "I've only lost my arm, not my brain" would help my cause one iota.

It seemed amazing to think that the air ambulance that rescued me was based not far from my home. Colin and I both felt the need to give something back so we contacted them and were duly interviewed and accepted as volunteers. Having met the doctor while I was in hospital I wanted to meet the rest of the crew and a date was arranged for us to visit the base. On the way Colin asked if I was okay – why shouldn't I be? I felt a bit excited but otherwise very calm and relaxed. Sadly the paramedic was not available on the day but I could meet the pilot. We waited in their reception area and shortly after our arrival a door opened and in walked a guy dressed in flying gear – it was he. I walked towards him to shake hands but instead flung my arms round him and burst into tears. Where did all that emotion come from, I wondered – well what can compare with hugging and being hugged by a man who played a massive part in saving your life?

The February day of our visit was mild, bright and sunny so after a much needed coffee and chat we went out to see the helicopter. What a beautiful, friendly machine, just a place of work for a few and yet capable of evoking a vast range of emotions for so many.

During the summer of that year the Kent Surrey and Sussex Air Ambulance held an open day at their base. We attended with a large crowd of friends; how wonderful it felt that so many of our friends were supporting us as well as the air ambulance. It was a big affair with lots of attractions including helicopter rides and I could not wait to book myself a flight.

While a friend and I joined a queue for food I spotted a chap in the familiar red flying outfit. No sooner had I told my friend that I wished I could tell him that one of his colleagues had helped save my life when I realised he was walking towards me. "Excuse me, m'am," he said, "I believe I was on duty when ..." Yes, he was my paramedic! How good was that? Now I had met the whole crew.

As volunteers for the Surrey Sussex and Kent Air Ambulance Colin and I have the opportunity to attend interesting events, raising awareness and funds for the charity and the bit I like best is meeting and talking to the most fascinating people.

We attended a wonderful concert in Guildford Cathedral and when our meeting and greeting duties were over we took our reserved seats in the audience. During the interval I discovered that the couple I was chatting to were the parents of a young man also rescued by the KSSAA. Their son's amazing story sounded familiar, as I had read it on the charity's website. He had been pronounced dead at the scene of the road accident but despite this the helicopter doctor insisted on attending to him. The young man survived and the doctor in attendance was the same doctor who attended to me.

"I always support them," said a man as he donated at our stand at the Surrey County Show in Guildford one summer. "I work at the Royal London Hospital." Of course we had a chat and he said he thought he had seen me before. Indeed he had; it turned out that he was the medical photographer. We joked about me being denied sight of my pictures to spare me any distress and he said I could contact him and see them.

Hours spent standing outside a supermarket might seem unbearable to some but wear an Air Ambulance tabard, hold a collecting tin and watch and listen as life's rich tapestry unfolds before you. It's like a scriptwriter's dream to see how some of the general public present themselves for a trip to the shop; also the way they react to the charity collector. Some people immediately approach, coins at the ready, and tell you what a wonderful organisation the Air Ambulance is. Others give coins to small children to donate, some apologise for only having small change. No matter how little or how much is given it is always gratefully received and I never fail to thank them for their support. As volunteers we are told that just a pound's worth of bubble wrap can save a life. Very few pass without some behavioural trait when they don't wish to donate. Often the mobile or watch has to be checked, speed is of the essence, the keys have to be hunted, the imaginary friend looked out for, the list is endless. The main attraction for me, after raising funds and awareness for this wonderful charity, is chatting to interesting people. It is incredible how much one learns from complete strangers, while holding a collecting tin.

Of all the memorable events while collecting at supermarkets the two that stand out most in my mind both happened on the same morning. A bright looking young lad about ten years old came and stood confidently in front of me. "Can you tell me what this charity does and where does the money go?" I was very impressed by his intelligent enquiring attitude. Some children are handed money to give away without knowing why or where it was going. I explained how the air ambulance always saves time and often saves lives by having a special doctor on board who could deliver the Accident and Emergency service to the patient at the scene of the accident rather than waiting till they arrive at hospital, and all the money collected goes towards keeping this service available. The young lad was very attentive showing great interest; he then donated the money he had been holding. I then said I would tell him something very special; the air ambulance had rescued me and saved my life. He looked at me incredulously as I assured him that I would not be there had it not been for the air ambulance. His young face was full of wonder and I'm sure we will both remember our meeting. As he returned to a car parked nearby I noticed the driver's window was open. I hurried over and spoke to the driver; yes he was the boy's father. I congratulated him on having a lovely son, the first child I had met to take such a serious interest in the charity. The driver gave me a lovely smile and a thumbs-up sign before driving away. It was a special moment and then I realised it had been parked in a disabled bay.

Store collections are rarely boring, especially this one where the trolley attendant chatted to me while still conscientiously doing his job retrieving trolleys and helping people who did not have a pound coin, or if they did have one it was stuck in the trolley. He was a very helpful chap, well known to many of the regular shoppers. I would guess that he might have found this employment following an illness or accident as he told me of his days involved in the development of silicone adhesives; he certainly knew a lot about them. He also had a very interesting sense of humour, definitely verging on a shade of black, I would say. A leaflet he retrieved from a trolley turned out to be someone's funeral service, complete with one picture of the deceased and another of a family group. The service had taken place about fifteen months previous and inside the card were two long poems both of which he proceeded to read to me, with a slant towards comedy but without being too irreverent.

When he next returned from his trolley retrieval he obviously felt confident enough to ask me questions:

"Did you get a free helicopter ride then, for being a volunteer?"

"No way! Well, actually I did, but I don't remember anything about it"

"Did you lose your arm in an accident then?"

"Yes, and the air ambulance rescued me."

"Traffic accident was it?"

"No, it wasn't."

"What was it then?"

"Well, I'm afraid you'll have to wait till my book comes out!"

"Oh, writing a book are you? My Dad started writing a book, he thought it would be nice for us to know all about his life before he died. Pity he died before he finished the book."

Having shared this family gem with me, he strode off across the car park to collect more trolleys. After a while the trundling sound of a snake of linked trolleys preceded his return. Giving his 'snake' a final shove, he raised his arms triumphantly. "I've got it," he said, "you stepped out of the helicopter and waved!"

Being able to drive is a huge factor in personal independence and I needed that independence back. I arranged for a driving assessment to check my ability to cope behind the wheel again. The assessment was very comprehensive and lasted all day with many aptitude tests to undergo before actually sitting in a real car. A test in a simulated car recorded my reaction times to a continuous random sequence of traffic light instructions. I was given a passage of text to read and instructed to count how many times a certain sequence of letters appeared. I had a recorded passage of text to listen to and count every time a certain word occurred. I was shown flash cards in fairly quick succession and had to make judgements as to the exact location of printed dots in relation to lines on the cards. I then had to read the text passage again, this time whilst listening to a story, and count a different letter sequence in the text.

Unaware of how good or bad I was doing, I carried out all these tests quite relaxed and calmly; it seemed so amazing to me that I could cope with this so comfortably when months before I couldn't even read the newspaper. I was given a print out of my test results and when they were explained to me it appeared that I had achieved above average scores throughout; I was thrilled and astounded.

Having completed the intensive day of tests, at last I got behind the wheel and had a test drive with an instructor. The car was adapted with a knob on the steering wheel so that I could safely drive with one hand. It felt great to drive round the test area site with its pedestrian crossing, traffic lights and parking bays and even better when we then ventured out into the general traffic and I was still okay. I had never been a confident driver when away from familiar ground but now here I was, driving an unfamiliar car, somewhere I had never been before and I was enjoying it. What joy, I was okay to drive.

Just to make sure and give me more confidence, I booked two two-hour driving lessons with a specialist instructor in an adapted car. Some of my lessons involved driving in the dark, on single track roads and in areas I had not driven in before and again, in a different car. I could hardly believe how much I enjoyed my driving and what a morale boosting achievement it was for me.

My retirement present to myself had been a gorgeous silver Smart car and I had loved it. Its size belied the spacious feel when driving it. With black leather upholstery and air conditioning, it was my pride and joy. I still miss the novelty of my Smart car but for practical reasons it was exchanged for an automatic Mazda. I had a 'lolly pop' adaptation fitted on my steering wheel as I found this much more comfortable than the knob which made my hand feel cramped.

Slowly but surely life was getting back to some kind of normality. There would always be limitations to what I could do but if I couldn't work it out there would also always be a bit of help available when needed.

Realising my London to Brighton rides were over my Raleigh tourer had been replaced with a Brompton folding bike and Colin had one too. When we ventured to try a caravan holiday I insisted my bike went with us. We managed to have a successful, enjoyable short break in Wales and coped quite well in our caravan. I was really chuffed at this and I was able to ride my bike in the safety of the caravan site.

One thing I could not manage was being able to carry our cutlery and crockery in our bowl to the washing up facilities on the site. Colin did all the washing up so it didn't matter too much but I felt miffed that I couldn't do my share. When I saw a lady carrying all her washing up in a big blue bowl with a handle I had to talk to her and find out where I could get one. It turned out the lady had bought the bowl in her homeland of Switzerland.

Imagine my delight when a few minutes later the lady came to our caravan carrying the now empty blue bowl. She presented it to me as a gift and profusely refused any thought of payment. If that lady ever reads my book she will learn how invaluable that bowl still is to me several years on. It is basically my laundry carrier but with the handle over my arm it is possible for me to carry several items around indoors and still be able to open a door as well. That blue bowl is very precious as it also represents a symbol of generosity. That is something I had often encountered even before my accident. When I had cut up an old pretty blouse and made it into a border of miniature patchwork for a bed sheet, I found a fabric remnant on a stall at Godalming market. While I chatted to the stallholder and pondered whether the colour was right as a backing strip for my border he really surprised me by actually giving me the fabric. Another time I remember trying on a navy blue velvet top and skirt in a Godalming shop. The shopkeeper provided a large cotton, mottled blue scarf to use while changing, to put over my head and protect the garments from make-up. I purchased the outfit and asked the price of the scarf, I thought it was lovely and wanted to buy it as well. To my amazement he folded the scarf, put it in the bag and handed it to me – he was actually giving me the scarf.

The Swiss lady who gave me the blue bowl and I swapped email addresses and we were surprised to discover that her address started with blue window and mine started with blue moon. What were the chances of that happening? Maybe once in a blue moon!

On a visit to her local library with my daughter one day a certain craft book caught my eye. It included patterns for knitting toys and things and I had to have it. What a good job I had not thrown out all my knitting needles; I found the correct size, acquired some white wool and set about knitting a little bird for my granddaughter. With one needle under my left little arm I struggled and cursed a bit in distress and ended up without a bird but with a bad back. Later I tried again with one needle vertically held between my knees. After some trial and error I eventually succeeded in casting on and following the pattern. I knitted the two sides of the bird, sewed it up and stuffed it. Two little black beads were sewn on for eyes and a small diamond of pink felt was folded and stitched in place for a beak. Finally I sewed a pink loop of ribbon on the bird's back. Imagine the thrill I felt to see my little white bird hanging on my daughter's Christmas tree and displayed on Facebook.

I pursued my knitting skill and also knitted a jumper for my three year old granddaughter. It was a replacement for a similar garment I had bought at a hospital craft stall that unfortunately did not survive a washing machine experience without shrinking. It was a very simple T-shape so very easy to copy without a pattern.

While I had been in hospital I was unaware that a young lady in London who had suffered an unspeakable horror when acid was thrown in her face had started the Katie Piper Foundation. Fortunately my plastic surgeon was aware and he passed my contact details on to the Foundation. I was contacted in connection with being on Katie's TV show, Katie My Beautiful Friends. Although it seemed a very exciting prospect it was still early days in my recovery for that kind of exposure so I was quite relieved when I was not actually selected to be on the show.

It was, however, an introduction to the Katie Piper Foundation which in turn led me to discovering a psychotherapist who was to play an important part in my full recovery. She was featured in a newsletter I read where she was introducing her services. Her experience in counselling was impressive, she looked beautifully serene in her picture and above all she was offering eight free sessions to the first five women to contact her. Of course the financial saving was inviting but what impressed me most was the fact that she was offering eight sessions. Obviously a lady who appreciated the importance of continuity and building trust and I believed she would be able to help me. Although I seemed to be doing very well and feeling fine I could not ignore the fact that I had suffered a very serious episode requiring medical, physical and emotional care for a full recovery. I had always kept my NHS psychiatric appointments but never felt a true psychological benefit as I never saw the same person enough times to build up a rapport. Life seemed so good for me but I felt the need to sort out what had happened to me and solve the mental 'but' I heard in my head when considering how I really was.

Not really believing for a minute that I would be one of the first five callers, I rang the number anyway and left a message. My call was returned and I learned that one of the first five callers had dropped out so I could arrange my first appointment. My belief in her ability was well founded and my time with her was invaluable. She said very little and I had the indulgence of metaphorically laying out the jigsaw pieces of my life in front of me and putting them back together in the right place. After my third session I told Colin I felt like I was turning a corner. It was like a subtle gear change and I knew I was getting back on track. I mentioned this at my next session and suggested that it be my last, particularly as there were many others whose needs were far greater than mine. One more visit was recommended just in case I had overlooked anything. I hadn't and when asked how I was I could now truthfully answer that I was fine without any mental 'buts' in my head.

The benefit I derived from my sessions was beyond price. The fact that I had found this contact myself seemed to heighten my benefit and I was inspired to write the following lines to express my feelings:

I have the strength to face the past with honesty

The wisdom to live in the present with appreciation, and

The courage to face the future, no matter what.

How lucky am I? I even have my own philosophy!

---oOo---

CHAPTER XIII

Operations operations operations

It was a cold, dry December day when we had to make the trip to London for the first of my many clinic review appointments at the RLH. We had coffee with friends who lived in Marshall Road, near the station, and as we sat in their conservatory I noticed scaffolding around the house next door, I wondered what was going on there. Apparently the large Victorian house was being converted into four flats. Eventually we were to achieve our wish to live in Marshall Road again when we moved into the ground floor flat.

We left our friends' house and got to the station in good time for our train. I had always enjoyed a trip to London and for me this was no exception. I remember feeling so pleased to be dressed smartly, in my best winter coat, and getting out and about again. As we approached the platform, however, Colin drew back, reluctant to enter the station. I confess this came as a bit of a surprise, because I was feeling so positive about our trip, so I thought Colin might feel the same.

We set off on all our train journeys to London from the next station up the line so we never returned to the scene of my accident. However, when Kelly (my hospital patient friend) was coming to stay for a few days, she arrived at Godalming station. What better reason could I have to walk on that platform again than greeting a special friend, a friend I would not have if it hadn't been for the fateful event at that station?

Over the following years we made hundreds of hospital visits and Colin's confidence grew with every trip but he was always the anxious one concerned about me, while I enjoyed the pleasure of going out. The fact that we travelled by train had a positive effect on my sense of achievement – I could still do it in spite of everything that had happened. I knew I was lucky that flashbacks were not possible for me as there was nothing for me to remember.

As I progressed and my wounds improved, regular appointments to dressings, hand and scar clinics gave way to appointments with consultants to discuss various reconstruction options.

"It's amazing what they can do these days." Who hasn't uttered these words? It seems so simple when you see the finished article but there is always a long time span and a lot of hard work before reaching that point. As it was with my right ear, stage one was a skin grafting operation. My neck was the donor site and skin was grafted behind the site of my ear in order to enlarge a suitable area for Branemark implants to be sited to eventually support my prosthetic ear.

Weeks later when the grafted skin was stable enough I had another operation for the implanting of three metal pins around my ear hole. Several weeks later another operation was performed to expose the pins and place magnetic caps in place. When everything was healed and ready, impressions were taken of the area as well as of my left ear. A mould was made, then a model, and several visits later I was presented with my new right ear. Oddly enough, it didn't seem strange to see the 'full frontal' view of my ear – that's how I saw other people's ears anyway.

Meanwhile, I was having appointments at Morefields Eye Hospital where a prosthetic eye was being made for me. The route to this procedure began with impressions of my eye socket and photographs of my left eye. Appointments were made for me at various stages of construction to check on progress and fit. This prosthesis was to be attached with glue. Eventually I saw my new eye. I'm a lady who can actually look herself in the eye! I couldn't help thinking there seemed to be a humorous, slightly theatrical element entering my reconstruction.

"If I could have only one thing back, it would be my hair." I remember saying this to a fellow patient while I was still in hospital. The loss of my little finger was a nuisance, the loss of my ear meant my glasses wouldn't fit straight, the loss of my eye was inconvenient, the loss of my arm was frustrating, but the loss of my hair was most distressing.

A wig was the obvious first suggestion. I had an appointment with a hospital department supplying wigs to ladies who had lost their hair mainly from cancer. Reminiscent of the fun trying on 'Beatle' wigs in the sixties, there was an element of entertainment attached to trying on wigs; I could be a brazen blonde, a riotous redhead or a bewitching brunette. In the end I settled for a mid mouse-brown; I didn't want it to look too obvious. Whether it was obvious or not I felt I would never truly know. I don't think I could tell anyone their wig was anything but amazing so how could I expect others to tell me? Whilst the wig made me feel slightly better in public it unfortunately sapped my confidence in certain situations. Getting into a car, sitting in a theatre or café I always felt worried that my wig would get dislodged or caught on someone's bag moving behind me. This had been known to happen and, of course, I then had a situation where I wanted to put it straight and check in a mirror; not easy with only one hand.

I did some internet research on hair transplanting. Surely the thick hair on a proportionately small, undamaged area of my scalp could spare some roots to be transplanted at the top. Thin hair would be better than no hair. Excited with the knowledge I had gained I made my suggestion known to my plastic surgeon. He listened sympathetically and explained that my grafted scalp did not have sufficient tissue, etc to support hair roots. Just my luck, not enough top soil.

All was not lost, however; there was an alternative. A procedure I had never heard of called tissue expansion was explained to me. Balloon type bladders could be inserted under the hair bearing skin on my scalp. They would have valves where a saline solution could be injected at regular intervals over the following months to stretch the skin. When the area of skin was sufficient, the bladders would be removed and the skin, together with the hair roots, would be taken up and over to replace my grafted scalp. The effect would be similar to the transplants in that it would be thin hair but, as I have said; better than no hair.

To me, this was a no brainer and I wanted to go ahead with tissue expansion. The only downside, it seemed, was having two balloons in my head, which would be expanded until I looked like Mickey Mouse. I thought this was a small price to pay and decided I would just put a scarf on my head when travelling to London for my fluid top-ups every two or three weeks. Very few of my friends shared my view and whilst Colin supported my decision I knew he was concerned about it.

I had the operation and two bladders were inserted under my scalp. Three weeks later we went back to St Bartholomew's Hospital for my first top-up. So far so good. By the third visit things were going swell, and my bladders were swelling nicely. Sleeping comfortably was getting a bit tricky but it wouldn't be forever.

Then one day the area at the top of one bladder began to sting. It gradually got worse and the discomfort seemed to be spreading; it felt like I had put my head in a bees' nest. I rang the hospital and it was decided that I should attend for them to inspect my head. We duly travelled to London on a Friday and on inspection there was nothing obviously wrong and no infection present but it was decided to drain some of the fluid out of the bladder to reduce the pressure. If this did not solve the problem I should return to their clinic on Monday. I spent the weekend taking painkillers which did nothing to relieve my agony and now I had yellow stains on my pillow and sticky stuff in my hair.

Needless to say, we returned to the hospital on the Monday morning. This time an examination of the site revealed a leak through my scalp, which had now become infected. The saline solution had apparently been leaking under my skin before leaking out – talk about pouring salt on an open wound. I was immediately admitted as an inpatient and operated on urgently to remove the bladders.

I stayed in hospital for five days, Monday to Friday, a midweek city break. It was wonderful that Kelly, my friend and fellow patient from The Royal London Hospital, was able to pop across town and visit me. It was also during this stay that I again heard the harpist playing her harp in the ward. She had played so beautifully whilst I was in the Royal London Hospital, we chatted and she played a request for me; it was Paganini's Variation on a Theme.

Once again I looked like a Dr Who extra with a tube sticking out of my head to drain the wound. It remained in place for the whole of my stay and its removal was the last procedure before I was discharged. My whole stay had been okay and all I had to contend with was the shattering of my hope of having hair. I had been fed and watered, well looked after and pain free – until the drain was removed. The agonising pain as it was pulled, albeit as gently as possible, from my head was a nasty shock that I won't forget.

I admit I was very disappointed that my tissue expansion had to be aborted; in fact I felt devastated; now I would never have hair. Then I heard that just because it failed the first time didn't mean it couldn't be tried again, maybe this time next year I thought. Little did I realise that another amazing option to solve my lack of hair was on the cards for me and I didn't have to wait too long for it either.

Shortly after this I had an invitation to a Katie Piper Foundation workshop in London. I wasn't sure what this would involve but agreed to attend. Colin travelled with me and full of anticipation we made our way to the workshop address in Hammersmith. As I walked up the stairs a friendly young lady said hello. It was Katie, what a lovely surprise! I didn't know for sure that she would be there. She said that I could have a choice of treatments; make-up, hair or nails, etc. It sounded wonderful but I explained my injuries and that I had lost most of my hair so I wasn't sure what they could do for me. Immediately she replied that they could probably help with my hair loss. Whatever did she mean? Did I hear correctly? Yes, I had heard correctly and very soon after this I had a consultation arranged with the amazing Lucinda Ellery at her hair loss clinic in Hammersmith, in fact at the same address where the workshop had been held. We discussed the treatment Lucinda said I could have and she drew a simple sketch of a hairstyle. She showed me a photograph of a lady sailing on a boat with her medium length hair naturally blowing in the breeze. That lady had the Intralace system and it looked amazing but I could not believe I would ever be in that position. Yacht or not I wasn't bothered about being on a boat, but I wished I could have hair like that. Can you imagine how I felt when I learned that there was a permanent solution for me? I was blown away and filled with joy.

Just like Cinderella's my wish came true and I did have hair like that. Very soon after my consultation I spent a very long day at Lucinda's Consultancy and had an Intralace system fitted. Colin was brilliant and somehow managed to pass the day waiting for me. The décor and ambience was far removed from any clinic I had ever known. Everything was designed with comfort and indulgence in mind. It did actually take all day, but what a day. As well as flicking through magazines I had personal access to a laptop and could even choose from a list of films to watch. I chose the Devil Wears Prada and loved watching the film even more than reading the book. A rare purchase for me, I had bought the book on my retirement to read en route to New Zealand.

It was a day I will never ever forget. Can you imagine how it felt to have a full head of hair that I could feel and brush? It was another occasion when I was completely at the mercy of my emotions and I cried and cried with joy. I struggle to describe my feelings and I could hardly take in what had happened. Imagine being given the best treat of your life, then turned upside down and spun around. Yes, it was real, I hadn't had a dream, it was really mine to keep. Now I wake up every morning with hair, I go swimming every week with hair and I shampoo my hair as normal. I love it when I can feel my hair on my cheek and when it blows naturally in the breeze. I am so lucky.

I had no problem in giving my permission when asked if my before and after photos could be used by the Foundation in their literature and on their website. Even more exciting was seeing my picture on the Katie Piper page of *Now* magazine and reading the text saying Katie thought I was one of the most inspirational women she had met.

I was so excited and couldn't wait to show my Plastic Surgeon when I had my next appointment with him. He was also obviously very disappointed about my tissue expansion being abandoned but now I had something even better. How grateful I was to him for passing my name to the Katie Piper Foundation.

The Kent Surrey and Sussex Air Ambulance saved me, the Royal London Hospital staff gave me my life back and the Katie Piper Foundation 'put the icing on my cake'.

Although both my prosthetic eye and ear looked a good representation of the real thing, unfortunately they did not improve my confidence as I had expected. In fact I felt more self-conscious when I was wearing them. I also had issues with the glue; it was like giving it to a two year old. However careful I was, I invariably got sticky fingers, making it difficult to let go of the glue pot, not to mention positioning my eye.

I was very pleased when my surgeon referred me to another technician at another hospital for prosthetics with "more life". Another lengthy round of appointments for impressions and photographs finally resulted in a new prosthesis. The new model incorporated both the ear and the eye in a single prosthesis. Whilst the ear section just clipped on with the magnets, the eye part still required gluing in place. It was a big improvement but I still found coping with the glue a sticky predicament.

Self-assurance was also a bit of a problem. Remarks like "Oh, you're wearing your eye. Isn't it wonderful what they can do?" didn't convince me that it was wonderful so, of course, I tended to think it wasn't. My daughter gave me the benefit of her immediate honest reaction: it was horrid! Interestingly enough that did not really upset me because I had learned that loved ones often find it unbearable to accept fundamental changes to their nearest and dearest. Of course, for her my new eye was an alien part of her Mum and not the real thing.

Although in some respects the new prosthesis was an improvement it didn't solve everything. I don't think my expectations were too high, I just really wanted to be able to cope independently with my own personal needs.

Then one day I had an idea. Anchoring my prostheses to the kitchen worktop with my little arm, and with scissors in my hand I cut off the ear segment. Yes. I performed a Van Goughectomy in my kitchen. It was magic; I could now easily fit my ear on the magnets and wear it all day every day, whenever I wanted, without any problem at all.

Are you following my train of thought? How wonderful it would be to have a prosthetic eye fitted the same way, on magnets. Questions were asked, more appointments, more discussions. Finally I had a scan to ascertain whether my eye socket had sufficient area of bone with a density capable of accommodating and supporting the implants. I also had 3D imaging of my scull. Bearing in mind this area had been extensively damaged and rebuilt, I felt cautiously optimistic.

Wonderful news awaited me at my next appointment. Implants were possible and a date was fixed for my operation to be carried out at Charing Cross Hospital. Even though I was told I might not have to stay in hospital, when the day came, I took my overnight things with me just in case.

I remember coming round from the anaesthetic and being in the recovery room. Then I was taken to a lounge area where Colin was waiting for me and tea and biscuits were being served to recovering patients. I was feeling surprisingly bright considering I had just had surgery under full anaesthetic and I was told I was okay to go home. On the way to Waterloo by taxi, then home by train it seemed incredulous that I had had an operation that same day. The best bit came the next morning when I was able to have a lie in and did not have to make the journey home.

My surgeon mentioned taking some of my medical photographs to Vietnam and I learned that he worked there for a children's charity. I felt very pleased to think that knowledge gained from my own surgical procedures might be helping disfigured children in a different part of the world.

As with my ear implants, many appointments followed before I was ready to meet my prosthetic eye maker again. I was a little wary, however, as I had to explain to her how my original eye prosthesis had become separated from the ear. What a wonderful lady, seeing the thick edge where I had cut off the ear – she not only made me a new eye but also a new ear with a feathered thin edge which fitted discreetly.

Fortunately my original eyeball could be re-used in my new prosthesis. Needless to say, it proved a much better exercise to fit it on the magnets but it was a bit worrying to discover it still needed gluing to my skin at the inner corner. Slightly less of a sticky problem but a slightly sticky problem nevertheless!

The tear duct in my right eye socket had been the subject of discussions and correspondence over several years. Skin had not grown over this moist area and attempts with silver nitrate to encourage healing had failed. Whilst it was something I could live with, it was something I felt conscious of and it was a bit of a nuisance when I wore my prosthesis. Lots of moisture would collect under the eye section of the prosthesis making the skin surrounding my eye socket red and sore. Eventually it was agreed to try skin grafting over my eye socket by taking skin from my left eyelid.

On the appointed day I fasted from 7.00am as instructed and had my last sips of water at 11.00am as instructed. We attended at the Royal London Hospital at 11.00am, and watched a full waiting room gradually empty as one by one patients were called for their surgery. By early afternoon we checked the situation and was told that I was not due to be called for a while so Colin went off to get some lunch, no point in him fainting from hunger. Mid-afternoon I was given a drink of water to stop me getting dehydrated; I guessed it was going to be late when I had my op. It began to get dark and there were only a few patients left. Soon the room was empty apart from Colin and I. We checked at the desk, I was still listed for an op. We walked the length and breadth of the room and round the perimeter, why hadn't I brought the Scrabble? By 7.00pm we had serious doubts that my surgery would take place that day. Eventually two exhausted surgeons still in their blue operating gowns came through the door to speak to us. They were so apologetic; one operation had taken much longer than expected and now they had run out of time. I accepted that frequent long waits, cancellations and rearrangements are virtually impossible to avoid in hospitals and always allowed a full day for medical visits anyway; if I have any free time it's a bonus.

A second appointment, arranged for a month later, was also cancelled because an urgent cancer case had arisen. My operation was far from being a matter of life or death, and anyway, I wondered how many cases I had disrupted when I had urgent attention from the huge trauma team when I was an emergency.

Third time lucky? Yes, all according to plan. Checked in at reception, only four hours in waiting room, during which I was called in twice for identification and medical checks. This was to be my first operation in the new RLH since I had been an inpatient in the old hospital six and a half years before. This was in my mind when I was asked the first question: "Where are you having your procedure today?" "Here, in this hospital," I clearly announced. The nurse looked at me; I'm not sure whether she was confused or amused "Where on your body?" she asked. Oh, of course, they need to be sure they have the right patient and I need to be clear about what I am there for. I curbed my desire to giggle and correctly answered that I was having skin grafting to my right eye socket.

Back in the waiting room it was a relief to share my faux pas with Colin and give him a bit of light relief. Eventually it was my turn to get gowned-up ready for my op. Colin came with me and placed my clothes in the bag provided, which was labelled and locked away for safety. Colin kept my watch and jewellery with him. What a novelty, no wheelchair this time, I actually walked to the operating theatre. Soon horizontal on a bed I was wheeled in to be anaesthetised. One of the staff quickly introduced herself to me, saying she had been on duty at a previous operation of mine more than six years before, but I'm afraid I did not remember her. As usual, there was a problem with fitting a cannula in the back of my hand, and eventually they gave up and it was inserted in my foot. While this was going on the operating theatre door was pushed open just enough for the surgeon to give me an encouraging smile and a wave. That was lovely.

The next thing I knew I was in recovery and heard that I would be taken to a ward. I was soon told to shift over to the right, onto another bed. I tried to open my eye for the first time and could not see anything but the blur of the light above me. This was what I had expected and slowly I could make out other blurred shapes of Colin and the nurses. My bag of clothes had arrived with me, so with Colin's help I slowly started to get dressed. "What do you think you are doing?" asked a nurse. "Getting ready to go home," I said. "Oh no," she said, "You are here for the night." So this time I got to have a night in town after all.

Before he left to catch his train home I asked Colin to pass me my handbag. "Where is it?" he asked. "I don't know, I can't see anything," I replied. "It must be here somewhere." Well, it didn't seem to be here, there or anywhere, so one of the nurses retraced our steps to where I had got changed, as if she didn't have enough to do. When she returned empty handed she very calmly said she needed me to carefully remember exactly what I had done since being in the waiting room. Frantically trying not to panic, I recalled at one stage, putting my bag on the floor by my chair. It *must* be in the room where I changed. This time Colin accompanied the nurse as she retraced the route again.

Still struggling to focus through my blurred vision, I felt quietly confident that my bag would be found. However, when Colin and the nurse both returned empty handed my tummy did a one hundred degree flip. OMG, what now?

Colin had to leave or he would not get home by midnight. Despite my concern I managed to stay quite calm and was concentrating on trying to see properly. Blinking was like having an inefficient windscreen wiper – sometimes the haze cleared a bit, only to return like a fog. I looked towards the nurse whom I felt had given me enough of her precious time, only to realise that she seemed familiar, surely I had seen her somewhere before? She repeated my name – yes, indeed we had met before. I was her patient in Treves Ward in the old Royal London Hospital six and a half years before.

What a delightful meeting, how lucky was I to have this lovely nurse taking care of me again. She could not believe it was me and how I had changed!

By now it was getting late and I had to settle down for the night. The amazing reunion had taken the edge off my concern for my handbag and I tried to sleep. After a while I heard footsteps in the ward coming towards me. All I could see was the dark blue blur of the nurse's uniform. Gradually as she drew nearer I saw a blur of green. My tummy lurched, my heart skipped a beat, yes it was my nurse with my handbag. She had gone right back to reception where my bag had apparently been placed for safety after I had left it on the floor, by my chair in the waiting room. Right at the end of her duty, that lovely nurse had really gone that extra mile for me and I slept well that night.

The next morning I was thrilled to discover another nurse who had looked after me in Treves Ward. She even remembered the occasion when my birthday cake with candles had set off the fire alarm in the hospital. It was wonderful to have a laugh together over that memory.

When my paperwork had been completed and I had been given painkilling medication to take home, I just needed my cannula removed from my foot so I could have a shower and get dressed. Amid the exciting news of my reunion with some of my previous nurses, another nurse removed my cannula. I stood by my bed gathering my towel and clothes before heading for the shower when Colin called out to watch what I was treading in. I looked down and to my horror, saw red sticky footprints on the floor. "It can't be me!" I exclaimed. "I haven't got a wound." But I had forgotten about the cannula, because I had not put my foot up after its removal – it was like an open tap and blood had been pooling on the floor by my bed.

A ten minute delay while I rested with my leg up soon sorted things out, after which I could at last get showered, dressed and ready to go home.

Not so fast! I asked if there were any more staff from Treves ward still in the hospital. Yes, they were in Ward 13C. Colin agreed; we couldn't leave the hospital without going up to the thirteenth floor. We took the lift and made our way to ward C. Indeed, there were staff who remembered me, including the Ward Sister. I reminded her of how good I thought she had been the time she removed a staple from my eye socket. We hugged and looked at each other disbelievingly. It was mutually so good for them to see how well I had completely recovered.

I was so excited to be able to tell them about the way my life had changed and been enriched and to thank them personally for all they had done for me. Having had operations in several different London hospitals, I was very pleased and it seemed very fitting that my last operation was booked in at the Royal London Hospital. It had also proved to be the most eventful by far, almost like a pantomime. I have nothing but good feelings for that establishment. Full of care and compassion, in my book, they really are 'the business' when it comes to medical matters.

My mind often returns, with thankful thoughts, to all those who had played a part in my survival and reconstruction. Not least of all, the Air Ambulance Doctor, how wonderful it would be to let him know how well I was doing since our meeting while I was still in hospital. I sent him a text and he replied; we arranged to meet at the Royal London Hospital where he was still based. I could hardly believe how I felt, not only did I want to see him again I wanted him to see me.

---oOo---

CHAPTER XIV

A life enriched

While it must have been a huge relief for Colin to have me back home, albeit with a few bits missing, I'm sure he still had fears about my wellbeing. He always travelled with me to attend hospital appointments, workshops or charity events – not only was it preferable, it was safer too, especially if there was anything to carry. Naturally as time passed our mutual confidence grew and we relaxed a bit more about going out.

As I got stronger and fitter I sometimes went out with friends or would meet up locally for a coffee. On these occasions Colin would ask me to ring and let him know that I had arrived safely and when I was leaving. Of course I always did so but hated doing it because when the phone was connected I always had an image in my mind of him being alone at home with the phone ringing and was he wondering if it was the police on the line.

It seems strange that the following event that happened several years after my accident should have such a profound effect on me.

Buzzzzzz: our door bell rang one December evening in 2014. Fully expecting it to be our neighbour from upstairs, I confidently opened our door into the communal hall. There was no one there, I stepped out to see who the caller could be. It wasn't very late but it was dark, and I felt grateful for the window in the door to our porch so I could see who was there before I opened the door. I gasped as my breath involuntarily caught in my throat; I could see black with lots of 'bits' and a hat. A police uniform materialised right in front of me, through the glass. A huge gulp of air gushed up to my throat, trapping my daughter's name on my lips. "It's not bad news, it's ok." I heard these words, heaved a sigh of relief and opened the door.

The man of the law was correct, everything was ok, he was just house checking. I returned to our hall, Colin was there and suddenly I felt something deep within me. Sickening dread flashed through my brain and hit my stomach – Colin was there – I clung to him and as he hugged me I cried, with husky throaty sobs seeming to echo up from my tummy. I was alive, and I was safe, but I seemed to be living the impossible, a phantom event that I hadn't actually experienced. I could only imagine what Colin had gone through when the police rang our door bell more than six years previously when I had just gone out shopping and did not return.

My connection with the Katie Piper Foundation was proving extremely helpful and I have been very fortunate to attend several more workshops. As I got to know the extremely competent KPF staff and the other attendees, the full impact of the Foundation sank in. Feeling alone with your suffering is one of the most miserable things to happen to anyone experiencing scarring and disfigurement. Facial scars have a huge fundamental effect and can take the longest to accept; they must surely be the hardest to come to terms with. Most of us can relate to the horror of a bad haircut or a facial zit being enough to make us not want to see anyone, or indeed be seen. In time we realise that hair grows and zits can disappear but we have to learn to live with our permanent scars. This might seem hard or even impossible but it is possible and the tougher the battle, the bigger reward that victory yields. The ability to enjoy life again, and the personal pride in achieving this ability, is very rewarding.

The benefits for burns survivors to meet together and be totally accepted for who they are while enjoying the kind of events that most of us only dream about are invaluable. I've enjoyed everything from a Park Lane Spa pamper day to icing cupcakes and making chocolate truffles. All the events are very professionally run and very well organised. As well as social workshops the Foundation offers practical help in many ways. Not only with hair loss but also with medical tattooing, laser treatments and make-up camouflage, in fact everything possible to make life easier for burns survivors. Words almost fail me to describe how I think of Katie's Foundation and what it has done for me and many other burns survivors. From a terrible tragedy Katie has become an ambassador for generous inspiration.

I could hardly believe my eyes when I received an invitation in the post from The Rt Hon Jeremy Hunt MP requesting the pleasure of my company at the Key Supporters' Luncheon on behalf of the Katie Piper Foundation. I accepted and duly enjoyed dining in the Churchill Dining Room of the House of Commons in November 2012. It was another opportunity to meet very interesting people and I had no idea then that being a charity supporter would offer such rewards.

Before my accident I would have wondered what would be expected of me and felt nervous about attending a life-coaching course but when I was invited to attend such a workshop with the KPF I was excited and fired with enthusiasm. This course proved to be immensely valuable to me. I explored my newfound confidence and surprised myself with my coolness in being able to stand up at the front to answer a question. It also came as a surprise when the co-presenter of the course said she thought I would make a good speaker and we agreed to keep in touch.

What a blessing that I was given a leaflet when I left hospital for a charity called Let's Face It. Set up by Christine Piff, a lady who lost an eye from cancer; this charity helped and supported people with facial disfigurement. I was a bit worried when the possibility of having a prosthetic eye fixed onto a pair of glasses was being discussed. I could envisage quite a few problems with this arrangement so I rang the number on the leaflet and spoke personally to Christine who had started the charity. What a lovely lady and it was so helpful to talk to her. I had yet another surprise when she asked if I would like to write up my story for her charity's newsletter. It was incredible to read my own story when it was printed in the next newsletter.

We kept in touch and a couple of years later at Christine's suggestion I wrote an update to my story. When I reread my first instalment I immediately realised how far I had progressed in my recovery.

At about this time the lady who was the co presenter of the self-help course I had attended contacted me giving me my first opportunity into public speaking. It was a networking company's lunchtime meeting to be held in a lovely old pub. I was invited to join them for lunch and be the after-lunch speaker. Without a hint of nerves I duly delivered a ten-minute talk of my story and was very surprised and pleased by their response and positive feedback.

How timely that shortly after this I had an opportunity to join two other volunteers for the Katie Piper Foundation for a session with a public speaking coach in London. We had to prepare three presentations of varying lengths and perform them to each other for guidance and constructive criticism. It seemed amazing that this would have caused me lots of stress and sleepless nights at one time and yet now it was so good to enjoy this challenging project and revel in the creativity of it. I really looked forward to being a speaker for the KPF and couldn't wait.

It never occurred to me to fantasise about where I would speak and no doubt I would never have guessed my future venues. My first KPF booking was to speak to fourth year medical students at Southampton University Medical Faculty. I didn't go to university so a lecture theatre was new territory for me but I was not daunted;

I was excited. I took my seat and listened intently to the first speaker who was a burns specialist. I could relate to lots of his text and was fascinated by his gruesome pictures so much so that I momentarily forgot I was the next speaker. Again I had no nerves and enjoyed my delivery, receiving a very appreciative reception from the staff and students.

My next booking was not far from Southampton at a sports awards ceremony held by Valley Sports in Romsey. It was a super occasion and I spoke before the many awards were presented for sporting achievements. When my talk ended I started to leave the stage amid the applause when the MC told me to turn back and look at the audience. I did and could hardly believe my eyes: about two hundred people were on their feet giving me a standing ovation.

I could hardly believe it when I had a phone call from the KPF asking if I would like to attend as a speaker at a function in Liverpool. It was the NHS Tissue Services Review Day. I was thrilled to accept and Colin and I travelled to Lime Street station by train and stayed overnight in the Hard Day's Night Hotel just a few yards from the famous Cavern Club. It was our first visit to Liverpool and being right in the heart of The Beatles country was very exciting, not quite eclipsing the reason for our visit, however.

Opened in 2005, the Liverpool NHS Tissue Bank is the UK's largest and one of the largest in Europe. Their role is to retrieve, process, bank and supply human tissue grafts for use in surgery within the NHS. Many people who have heard of blood and organ donation may not realise the life saving importance of tissue donation after death.

The Review Day is an annual event for the dedicated staff of doctors, nurses, scientists, technicians and support staff to hear about the worthy results of their labours. My fellow speakers were a specialist transplant nurse and a heart surgeon who had very recently performed heart surgery on a newborn twin. The baby's father had travelled from Wales to be there and personally thank all involved in his son's survival. I was the third speaker and admit I felt humbled to tell my story following this technically amazing and emotionally moving account. I didn't have to study and work hard for my story; I have the easy bit of just telling what happened to me. I was just the recipient of incredible skills and a beneficiary of amazing services but I have since been told many times how significant it is to hear the patient's own experience.

My talk in Liverpool was the first time I thought of taking a couple of props with me. To demonstrate my craft skills I took my hairdryer bag and my granddaughter's jumper. I carried these items in a gift carrier bag with rigid sides so it was easy for me to transport and access the items when needed. On the way home as we took our reserved seats on the train to London I realised I had left the bag containing my props on the seat where I had been chatting to a fellow attendee on the platform. Fortunately an obliging guard on the train rang the station and confirmed identification of my bag and contents that were now safely in the custody of the station staff. They kindly agreed, in this instance, to send my bag to London on the next train. Actually it was quite opportune to have an hour's wait at Euston station as it meant we had time to have a sandwich and a coffee before taking possession of my props and continuing our journey.

My public speaking career seemed to have started on a high and I didn't think it could get any higher. Imagine how excited I felt when I had an opportunity to speak for the KPF for International Women's Day 8 March 2015. Five charities were to be represented at an event in the Chamber of City Hall in London. The venue was awesome and it was so lovely to see several Foundation friends in the audience who had come to support me. I was one of five speakers, all from very different walks of life, each telling of their life changing experience. My gratitude for what life had presented me with since my accident served to boost my confidence and incredible pride in representing the KPF charity. I truly understood the meaning of being empowered following my talk on this auspicious occasion.

It was brilliant to learn that Katie Piper was to be the fashion and beauty ambassador at the 2015 Ideal Home Show. When I had a call from the Foundation asking if I would like to be a model in Katie's diversity fashion show at the event I could think of nothing I would like better. I was one of eight models each with their own assortment of disability or scars proudly strutting their stuff to the beat of One Direction on several occasions during the exhibition.

Behind the scenes we had professional stylists, hair and make-up artists and co-ordinators; it was truly the most brilliant experience. Innovation feeds progress and the Foundation has certainly achieved huge advances for acceptance of human diversity.

2015 was also the twenty-fifth anniversary year for The Kent Surrey and Sussex Air Ambulance. A Georgian mansion in Kent was the venue booked for a summer tea party to thank volunteers for all their support and I was invited to be the guest speaker. A large marquee in the grounds was the elegant chandeliered setting for the afternoon tea and a harpist enhanced the occasion with her delightful music. It was another wonderful opportunity for me to extol the virtues of the charity and thank them for what they had done for me.

Imagine my surprise several weeks later when the charity asked if they could use my case in a presentation at another tea party for corporate sponsors to demonstrate the value of their support. It was another delightful afternoon tea at a beautiful venue and I was very impressed with the presentation, giving an up to the minute view of the incredible technology available to, and the sharply honed skill possessed by the helicopter crews. The audience attention was captured when the Director of Operations then gave an example of one of their missions.

The helicopter lifted at 10.42am to attend the scene. The patient was assessed as unstable. Treatment was administered to stabilise the patient. Time to deliver patient to Royal London Hospital was eight minutes. Despite multiple injuries and extensive high voltage burns the patient survived. At this point I left my seat at the table, joined the Operations Director and was introduced as the patient. I was so pleased to be the one able to demonstrate living proof of the value of the charity.

It had slightly puzzled me that I had not had a period of 'why me?' following my accident. I mentioned this when talking to the charity Managing Director and asked why me now? Why had I been the one honoured to have their case used and asked to tell their story. "Because you can," he replied. Yes, that's true, I thought, and it really sank in that all the appreciation and positive feedback I received after my talks was genuine and should be accepted by me in the sincere manner that it was given. I had frequently been told that I should write a book. Whilst I didn't really doubt my ability to write I did often have bouts of self-doubt. Is my story worthy, especially in the light of all the inspirational stories being told in the media?

When I wanted to ice skate I had no aspirations to be another Jayne Torvill so why should I worry about being compared with Jane Austen if I wrote a book? It just wouldn't happen so I should just get on and write... which is exactly what I am doing!

I'm afraid I couldn't hide my light under a bushel, I had to tell all about my exciting events. I just hope I haven't bored my friends and acquaintances too much. I gained a reputation locally for public speaking and received requests from The Women's Public Register, The Townswomen's Guild, the Women's Institute, the Mothers' Union and the Girl Guides. My story is always the same but my text is edited a little bit to make it appropriate for my listeners. Audiences have ranged in size from thirteen to more than two hundred and my venues from someone's sitting room to an impressive auditorium. I like to accept whenever invited to tell my story and never have I felt nervous.

I received a letter from a specialist clinical nurse who was part of the team involved in my reconstruction requesting my permission for him and a colleague to use my case and photographs in a presentation. I gave my consent and my story crossed the pond when they attended the Convention of the American Society of Plastic Surgical Nurses in Boston, Massachusetts and gave their presentation. As a footnote, they have now received a request to write it up for a journal. I will undoubtedly request a copy.

I joined the organisation called the U3A (University of the Third Age) for retired people and enrolled for ambling, scrabble and play reading. Ambling was wonderful, being taken out for a nature walk, learning about plants and birds, etc, while exercising in the fresh air and enjoying the beautiful local countryside. During one such walk we stood still in a wood and listened to a nightingale singing. I had not heard this beautiful birdsong since our early days in Godalming in the 1960s. Sadly it is now a very rare treat. Many years ago when the railway first came to Godalming the area was billed as the valley of the nightingales.

It was on another walk that I got chatting to a lady who told me her husband had lost both his legs and he attended a swimming club for the disabled. She gave me details of the club, I contacted my doctor and was duly accepted as a member. It had been many years since I had been swimming and I imagined paddling with one arm would mean I would go round in circles. The first thing I realised when I entered the water was how warm it was – what a pleasant surprise, no shivering and dipping to get used to the temperature.

Another surprise was that I could stay afloat and swim in a straight line. I swam breaststroke across the pool, apparently at a decent speed, and the instructor and physiotherapist escorting me suggested I try backstroke. I completed another pool width in a straight line and even faster. Where did that talent come from? Possibly all my years of cycling had given me strong legs. I became a regular Friday Swimmer and enjoyed swimming a modest twenty widths of the Olympic size swimming pool every week. I willingly agreed when asked if I would swim in the Club's gala thinking it would be a good opportunity for another exercise session. I confess I didn't think much more about it and was surprised when I discovered what a big event it was. A total of twelve clubs had entered, coming from the southeast area of the country as far afield as Windsor, Epsom and Hayling Island. No point worrying about it, I decided; I'd never been competitive anyway. My first event was a length of breaststroke and I was the only amputee; my opponents were seven youngsters with varying degrees of disabilities. Contestants were grouped together by their previously recorded times for swimming lengths. Enjoy your swim, I thought as I pushed off. Imagine my disbelief when I was told I had come first, I honestly thought they were joking. They weren't, it was true and I was presented with a gold medal. To date I have swum in four galas for the Club and now have five gold, three silver and one bronze medals.

When a friend rang one day inviting me to join her at a workshop for gospel singing at the local church, I took a little persuading. One thing I didn't do was sing, but I thought you don't need two arms to sing so I went. It was great fun and at the end of the workshop we gave a 'performance' in the church to a small audience who either knew about it or happened to be passing.

It transpired that a lady who had recently moved to Godalming from London missed her gospel singing so much that she was testing the water to see if there was enough interest in starting a local gospel choir. There certainly was and six years later I am proud to be a founder member of the Godalming Community Gospel Choir. We have given many performances including singing on the South Bank in London when we were one of the 30 choirs joining the London

Gospel Choir to celebrate their thirtieth anniversary. In the evening we all sang in the Festival Hall thus achieving the Guinness World Record for the largest gospel choir. What a claim to fame – and I was part of it!

The choir entered the BBC Gospel Choir of the Year competition and was one of the six finalists. The finals were being filmed at the Hackney Empire in London. I was not in the group singing but with Colin and my ex-hospital friend from Hackney we joined other choir members in the audience. GCGC did not win, but needless to say it was an amazing experience not to be missed.

At our next rehearsal evening I learned that a lady who had been an inmate at a women's prison when the choir sang there was also in the audience at Hackney and made herself known to one of the choir members. A life had been touched.

Once a year a group from the choir sing in a women's prison and I was very pleased when I was included to join them the next year. Not everybody gets the opportunity, or even wants to, enter a prison. I wasn't sure what to expect but knew it felt right to be there. I hope I get the chance to sing there again but I know the experience of that first visit could never be repeated. The women's participation, animation and expressions of appreciation were incredible. As I told the Chaplain, they were the best audience I had ever known. When the audience were leaving via the back of the hall, one lady changed direction and came forward. She passed a couple of choir members and wrapped her arms around me in a big hug. "Bless you," she said, "bless you for coming." "Bless you too," I replied. Another life had been touched and I will never forget that moment.

Another opportunity to tell my story came from a friend I made through the choir. My friend Hilary was now retired but had trained and nursed in the Royal London Hospital and asked if I would like to speak at a League of Nurses meeting. I was thrilled to agree to it and even more thrilled when one of my RLH surgeons agreed to give a presentation on head injuries prior to my talk. Having been a patient in the RLH it was very special for me to speak to an audience including so many ex-nurses from that hospital. Appreciation of the occasion seemed mutual and afterwards it was a pleasure to join them for lunch and have the opportunity to chat to some of them.

I told one lady that my next talk was to be representing the KPF at the South East Samaritans Conference. I told her of my regret at not joining the Samaritans years before and she confided that she was a Samaritan. She told me not to worry as I was being a Samaritan in what I was doing. It was so good to hear this.

A week later Colin and I were met at Tonbridge railway station in Kent and driven to the prestigious Tonbridge School. The school was the venue for the Samaritans Conference and we took our seats to hear the first speaker. She was an accomplished and eloquent speaker who spoke openly and honestly about her life struggles with eating disorders. I followed her with my story and then the last speaker was a young man called Junior Smart who told how he had turned his life around after a prison sentence for drug related gang crime in London and started a charity to help youngsters break the cycle of re-offending.

Once again I was in awesome company but I managed to dispel any self-doubt about the worthiness of telling my own story. After all, surely every true story stands alone not to be compared with another. It was definitely not a competition.

Seven years on and I can now hold my head high and face the past with honesty. Yes, I did suffer from a mental breakdown. At last mental illness seems to be getting more of the attention it deserves. Of all the illnesses that can befall human beings I can't help thinking mental illness to be one of the most frightening, to be suffered alone. Early symptoms can be kept as your secret and friends can be forgiven for thinking you need to take a break. As symptoms get worse the secret gets harder to keep so the desire to socialise gets less and less until isolation becomes an only friend. If you tell you may be stigmatised or possibly eventually sectioned and deprived of your freedom. If you don't tell you may be deprived of your life but your suffering will be over. What kind of choice is that!

Seven years might seem a long time for full reconstruction and recovery but in reality I've had seven wonderful years. The incredible awareness of surviving a life threatening accident has never left me and it feels like being a member of an exclusive club. In a low-key kind of way, each anniversary of my accident is a special day for me to give thanks for my life. I am so grateful that I can use my experience to help others.

My seventh anniversary was particularly poignant as it was also the tenth anniversary of the 7/7 London bombing so there were many reminders in the press and on television. It was also the year of my seventieth birthday on the seventh of September. What better opportunity to say a big 'thank you' to family and friends for all their support and friendship, so I decided to hold an afternoon tea party to celebrate the occasion. Everyone invited was requested to wear a hat and there were to be no birthday presents but instead donations were welcomed in the hatbox provided, to the KSSAA and the KPF. The theme of the day was giving thanks and to help the party go with a swing I booked a singer, Gloria Miller, a lovely lady I had heard performing at one of our charity events. She was wonderful, singing all the numbers Colin and I had specially chosen, including Simply The Best, The Power of Love, I Will Survive and Oh Happy Day. The sky was blue and the sun shone all day, it was a lovely event in beautiful surroundings, everything I could have wished for to celebrate being alive – I had a ball!

When booking our next Scilly Islands holiday we thought we might go in high season. It had been quite cool in our last visit in May so we decided that it would be worth the extra cost for a warmer holiday. A few dates were offered and I settled on 7 July. Not until Colin pointed it out to me did I realise that I had selected the anniversary date of my accident.

Here are a few of the many rewarding experiences I would not have had if I had not had my accident:

Meet so many incredible people

Move in circles I would never have entered

Be a charity volunteer

Have lunch at the House of Commons

Be a public speaker

Win medals in swimming galas

Be a fashion model at the Olympia Ideal Home Show

Attend workshops and functions

Sing in public with an amazing gospel choir

Write this book

I hope I have many more years of life to come and however tragic it may seem I do believe I am fortunate to have had a life experience that has shown me however bad it gets it definitely can get better. That experience has given me knowledge and a deeper understanding and appreciation of life.

I am really grateful that my parents had passed away before my accident but I can't help thinking that they would be proud of my life and achievements since my accident. "A blessing in disguise" was one of my Dad's many sayings. Whilst it may not immediately seem apt and the physical losses I sustained could no way be described as a blessing, I am certainly blessed with a wonderful life. I like to think that if he were here today Dad would feel confident enough to address the situation thus.

When there is a loss in one's life, be it retirement or bereavement, my suggestion for filling that void is to volunteer for a charity that is dear to your heart. Donate money if you want to but give your time; it's so easy for something you are passionate about and so rewarding.

I did just that and earned the rich rewards of giving, something far more valuable than receiving a monetary salary.

Was I in the wrong place at the wrong time or the right place at the right time? What did God or luck have to do with it? My rescuers came from the sky – was it fate? My medical team were the best in the business – was it skill? My support network was second to none – was it love? "Divine intervention" – was it God? I certainly don't know the answer and I don't think it matters either way. Whichever way you look at it I'm just eternally grateful that I had a valid return ticket.

CHAPTER XV

Recollections

Angela was a lovely, lively courier I met on a holiday in Northern Ireland. After a chat over coffee one day she asked to be included on my list of email addresses for when my book came out. She went further and suggested I ask some of my friends to write a memory of me. I decided to contact a few friends and acquaintances from before and after my accident, to write a paragraph about me. I requested complete honesty, warts and all! I sincerely hope that everyone who has contributed has also given me the compliment of complete honesty:

1. My first meeting on the Sunday night. You looked so elegant, tall with that natural style that works and the classic bob. So a really nice couple. It was only the next day that I noticed your arm. I didn't think much, maybe like, you were born that way. Then for some reason our paths crossed in the coffee shop at Mount Stewart. The three of us got chatting and at that point I got to hear your story. I remember your husband had such a clear memory of every detail of that day and his visits to the hospital after, it is amazing how the memory is

so sharp at a time of shock. My own husband had bad cancer when my youngest was two; I still remember every detail. I could have spent hours listening to such an amazing story, suppose it could happen to anyone going about their life, Lin, but in your case you are living proof of recovery and survival, that's . what was so amazing. I could not believe what I was hearing. Such an amazing story of bravery. You are a very strong, positive woman, a fantastic ambassador for anyone who will experience such trauma. Angela x

---o0o---

2. It was 1964 – I was sitting at my desk, biting into an apple when in walked this gorgeous willowy young lady who was to be the new secretary. Her desk was next to mine and we hit it off immediately. She said, "I've only been married for six weeks" – I replied "Oh we've been married for six years". In no time at all we arranged for our husbands to meet and the four of us got on like a house on fire. We regularly visited various pubs and went back to each other's houses to put the world to rights over cups of coffee. Pete gave Colin some driving lessons to start him off and one day Lin and I were sitting in the back of the car and I was moaning about my stockings being wrinkled (Nora Batty). She said, "I no longer have that problem", lifted her skirt to reveal a pair of TIGHTS, what a trend-setter. They were the first ones I had ever seen – In no time at all I hot footed it to the shops to buy some for myself. Colin worked at the Gomshall Tanneries and to repay Pete for his lessons he ordered two beautiful

dark brown sheepskin coats for us at a hugely reduced price – we were the trendsetters then as there were not many about at the time.

We have been friends ever since and whenever we meet we still to this day enjoy a jolly good laugh. Thank you for those years of valued friendship – love to you both – Pat & Pete x

---oOo---

3. I first met Lin back in the 1990s. I needed additional office staff and Lin joined my team. She soon proved to be a real asset and we become good friends. The company was going through change and this meant I needed Lin to take on more responsibility. She was more than capable but her real lack of self-confidence meant I spent a long time convincing her she was more than up to the challenge.

    The firm was eventually broken up and sold off and we all went our separate ways. Lin and I kept up the Christmas card ritual for the next 10 years. Then in 2009 I helped organise a reunion but Lin did not feel up to coming and facing everyone, it only being a year since her life changing accident.

    It was not until Jan 2016 that I finally got back together with Lin and her husband Colin. She was still the same lovely person I had known all those years ago but now there was a drive and self-confidence I had not seen before. Whether despite or because of the trauma she has gone through, Lin is living life to the full. God bless her. It is a privilege to call you my friend. John Martin

---oOo---

4. Lin and I go back quite a few years (I think back to 1995?). In fact, I got to know her through my husband as they worked for the same company in Godalming. She was a tall, slim lady always very elegantly dressed. We had just moved to Surrey, so everything and everyone around us was new. Lin was not shy, she seemed to know quite a few people and was involved in various activities. Tennis, table tennis, theatre, you could describe her as someone who liked the company of other people I think. She got my husband to join the tennis club and later they also played table-tennis, which I enjoyed too.

    When we bought our first house in Godalming, it turned out that our 90-year old neighbour was Lin's Dad! She came to visit him several times a week and also did his shopping. We gradually got to know the rest of the Woolmington family, Colin (or Mr Woolmington), Katherine, their daughter, and Lin's sister and brother-in-law. Lin seemed an outgoing person, always organizing something or other. I remember one year, our son was a baby, she organized a youth-hostelling weekend, for a group of friends, none of whom we knew. It was a great weekend, with lots of walking, laughs and even some singing in the evening, after a very nice dinner prepared by Lin and Colin (oh yes, I remember the bread and butter pudding, Colin, with custard, of course!).

    Some time later my husband got a new job and we moved to a nearby village and so we got to see each other less often. We kept in touch, mainly by phone or the occasional chat over a cuppa. Then one evening, it had been a while since I last heard from the Woolmingtons, I decided to give them a ring. Colin answered the phone. There was a big silence. Then Colin said: 'I'm so sorry. You haven't heard the news. Lin is in hospital in London.' In fact, she had been for almost 2 months. Colin told me the story, that Lin had been airlifted from the railway line, that she had life-changing injuries and she would be in hospital for quite a bit longer. Colin also told me then that Lin had been suffering from depression, but that no one had realized how bad it was. All this was such a shock to me, I just couldn't believe it. How could something like this have happened? Not to Lin, such an outgoing person, always ready to help others. I cried all night in the kitchen.

A little later I went to visit Lin in hospital. I was a bit nervous because I didn't know what to expect really. I took a box of chocolates and a bottle of wine. I went into the room and saw Lin, her face all bandaged up. Colin was sitting next to her. There I stood holding my box of chocolates! Lin could hardly move her mouth. Then I noticed she also had an arm missing. I tried not to be in shock too much, it was so overwhelming. Lin made it easier for me because she had such a happy expression on her face. Despite all her terrible injuries and the fact she had been stuck in a hospital bed for three months, she said she was 'lucky' to be alive!

From then onwards I have always seen Lin in an upbeat mood. She seems to have adapted this new 'don't worry, be happy!' philosophy. She does so many things, it is impossible to sum them all up (swimming, singing, sewing, fundraising, to name but a few). Trying to meet up with her is not easy as she is always busy doing something or going off somewhere. She is very good with her hand (and feet) too. I am not very good with a sewing machine, but somehow I got myself into making some costume bits for my daughter's Christmas ballet show. I didn't know where to start. I mentioned it to Lin so she invited me over and showed me how to put a top together, sitting on the floor and handling the fabric with one hand and a foot. Amazing. I think she also made her own curtains and some gorgeous bunting for my kitchen and my daughter's bedroom! However, to me personally, her greatest achievement is her positive thinking. I never really knew that Lin had been through a period of serious depression. Which just shows that you can hide a lot of things. Depression is not something that is talked about easily. It is an invisible illness that can cause a lot of damage and it takes quite a bit of confidence, determination and – not to be forgotten – support from others to get through.

In short, I think Lin has really turned her life around and through the months and years after her accident she has discovered qualities she was never even aware of. I'm sure she had never thought of becoming a public speaker and still, she has given numerous talks in front of a variety of audiences (from medical students to WI ladies). Through her disabilities Lin has had the opportunity to meet various people who have made a big impact on her life (Katie Piper and the staff of the Surrey and Kent Air Ambulance spring to mind). She has grasped these opportunities to do something with them and to become an inspiration for other people. She has certainly become an inspiration to me. I would like to wish her all the best with her future plans (and she's got quite a few lined up) and hope to be her friend for a long time to come. With all my love, Els.

---oOo---

"There are no constraints on the human mind, no wall around the human spirit, no barriers to our progress except those we ourselves erect."

Ronald Reagan.

5. The first time I met Lin, she had been brought to the Emergency Dept of the Royal London Hospital as a trauma call. What I saw was a woman who had sustained such terrible injuries and at the time, I wondered to myself, even if she survived what her future would be like, what would she look like? How would she deal with her life now that it had irrevocably changed? How would her family react?

    I never thought that I, amongst other healthcare professionals would be asked to walk beside her on her slow, eventful and often painful progress which involved many periods of reconstructive surgery at the Royal London Hospital.

    Over the years of managing complex wound care issues I often hear people remark that life is never easy, yet I witnessed with my own eyes the strength of the human spirit regaining itself as she battled through and won her place back as a wife and mother. To see her inner self and personality come through as she finds her new role as an ambassador for others who have, and often still are, struggling with traumatic and life changing injuries has been a truly rewarding part of this journey. Daren Edwards MBE RGN Clinical Nurse Specialist Plastic Surgery. The Royal London Hospital, Barts Health NHS Trust

---o0o---

6. Dear Linda, Sharing with you my thoughts of how well you did in your journey. You have been through a lot since your accident but managed to pull through. This with your sense of perseverance and patience helps you face all the treatments you have undergone. You have had so much support from your family and your husband Colin has been without doubt the one driving force in your long and frightful recovery. There were times I noticed you attended the clinic feeling hopeless but you managed to pick yourself up. Not a lot of patients can do the same as what you did.

    Seeing you now so active and involved in charitable organizations, helping those who may benefit from your experience such as other people, their families and friends, carers and the hospital teams is truly a great success for you considering the traumatic experience that you went through.

    Lastly, indeed I learnt a lot of experience looking after you and this surely will benefit me in looking after other patients too. I would like to take this opportunity to wish you all the best. Best Wishes.

Yours sincerely, Lyn, Sister F. Selim, Scar Management Clinical Nurse Specialist, Royal London Hospital.

---oOo---

7. I met Lin in 2008 whilst I was recovering from some reconstructive surgery, a year and a half after I was involved in a near fatal road traffic collision whilst cycling to work in London. I was on a ward at the Royal London Hospital, when a rather sad and afraid woman was wheeled in. Lin said very little at first, but it was very apparent that whatever had happened to her, it was incredibly serious. Sitting opposite one another on the ward, day in day out with little to do gave us the chance to start to get to know one another slowly. By the time I was ready to leave a number of weeks later, Lin had confided the details (at least what she could remember) of what had happened to her. I was shocked and confused! Here was a very attractive, able woman, in the prime of her life, surrounded by a loving family, yet she had felt so desperate that she hadn't been able to face continuing.

Over the years I have become (at least I would like to think!) a close family friend. I have got to know Lin, her husband Colin and her daughter Katherine well. Lin made a remarkable recovery after the first incident and I was amazed and proud to see how well the family had united and the lust for life that Lin seemed to have again! Little could I have foreseen what was about to happen again in 2016.

I was at home in France when I received a call from Katherine. It quite literally floored me. It had happened again – I hadn't spoken to Lin for a number of months but had been in contact more recently. I was literally kicking myself: how had I missed the signs? I knew she seemed down, but surely not that bad. I recall her having a wonderful day in London planned, she had just spent some time with her daughter and grandchildren – everything seemed so normal. But that's the thing with mental illness. Sufferers become very good at hiding their true feelings, from their friends, their families and even themselves. I knew she had hit rock bottom and there was only one way she could go from there – up. I'd seen her do it before and I knew she could do it again, no matter how tough it was going to be or how long it was going to take this time.

I visited Lin not long after she had been moved to the Royal Surrey hospital, in November 2016. I could see clearly just how low she was in herself and how tough her recovery was going to be. I'm pleased to say that, although it did take time, it wasn't too long before this vibrant and tenacious lady was back on her feet (or should I say foot and prosthetic) and fighting to enjoy life once again.

When I saw her most recently I can certainly say she's fighting fit, upwardly mobile and enjoying what life has to offer again. We never know what hand life is going to deal us, or how we're going to react and there will always be ups and downs. One thing I'm certain of is that it takes real guts to get over something like Lin has endured; once let alone twice. I know that there's guilt and shame associated with what's happened, but I for one would like Lin to feel proud. Proud that she's had the courage to take life by the balls again, proud that she has a wonderful supportive husband in Colin and proud that they have raised a daughter who has been there for her Mum and her Dad through all of the ups and the downs. Our friendship means the world to me and I feel very privileged to be able to call this remarkable lady, my dear Lin, a friend. Kelly xx

POST SCRIPT

I thought my story was finished but in 2016 an event occurred that brought about a feeling in me that had huge repercussions.

Our dear friends Pat and Pete had often said that they wanted to die together. No doubt this would apply to lots of couples after many years of marriage. Pete had been seriously ill for some eighteen months and Pat had made an amazing recovery from a double mastectomy a couple of years previous and she still seemed full of life. Early in the year Pete's health was giving real cause for concern and Pat asked us to cancel a proposed visit.

Then one morning we read an email from Pat that she had sent late the previous evening. She was saying goodbye, instructing us not to try and save them and that they had left Pete's mobility scooter to Colin who had been diagnosed with Parkinson's.

This was a huge emotional shock and we were not prepared for it. When Colin and I recovered some composure we wondered what we should do, if anything. Who else knew what we knew? Surely we weren't the only ones. I didn't want to be the one to ring the police so we finally decided to show the email to the community policeman on duty in our local council offices. His first reaction was to question us with a 'why didn't you try and stop them' kind of attitude. Needless to say this made us feel very uncomfortable but he soon realised we were not part of their plan. He rang Guildford Police station and a policewoman consoled me on the phone while her colleagues attended the scene. Later in the afternoon two policewomen called at our home to inform us that their colleagues had found both our friends dead on their arrival.

Pat and Pete had been part of our lives for more than fifty-one years, ever since we married. We received a reply from a relative of Pat's to our condolence message, which, although thanking us for our message, added hugely to my pain: "Why did we pre-empt things by calling the police who had to break in, there was no need ...?". We were not privy to any plans, what did she expect us to do?

This whole occurrence certainly triggered some irrational thoughts and emotions in me: Did my past experience give them the idea? I felt an element of guilt. They had escaped any indignities of old age that may have befallen them. I felt an element of envy. Above all there was the grief of losing two very good friends whom we had spent a Christmas with and holidayed with, not to mention the wonderful sense of humour we shared!

Several months later we visited our friends' home and the mobility scooter was put in our car boot for us. Memories of many happy previous visits were very strong as was the pain of grief. When we got home the realisation that neither Colin nor I could remove the scooter from our car really hit me like a kick in the stomach. I suddenly felt completely useless, how on earth was I going to help Colin if his Parkinson's condition worsened and how could I look after myself without his help or be of any help to our daughter and grandchildren? This all became a huge issue to me, and all my other every day concerns gradually began to get out of proportion. I became so anxious I could not sleep, panic attacks plagued me, I could not eat, my voice changed and my mobile phone and laptop became completely alien to me, I was actually scared of them!

All these feelings were horribly familiar – I had been here before. Depression had returned. I tried hard to deal with things but knew

I was losing the battle. I derived no pleasure from going out socially and didn't really want to see anyone. I knew Colin, my daughter and my friends were worried about me again. I could not hide anything, my voice gave away that something was wrong as soon as I spoke, especially on the phone.

"Seek help," I said to myself so I rang the number on the card I had been given by my psychiatric doctor. I had kept this card in a safe place for more than eight years knowing it was my lifeline in case of emergency. I tried to make an appointment but was told the doctor was on leave for two weeks, what a blow that was. But after a few days I thought I would ring again and get an appointment arranged for after her return. Another shock was in store when I learned that I would need a referral from my GP as I had not seen her for more than two years. That was not all; I could no longer see my original psychiatric doctor as I was now above the age of 65 and no longer in the age group she dealt with. In my fragile state this news was like a door being slammed in my face.

I tried to make an appointment to see my GP. He was not available so I saw another doctor who I had not seen before. I related my whole history of depression and what had happened to me, the doctor listened sympathetically and I felt she understood my situation. After six years on medication and feeling good, with my doctor's approval I had been weaned off pills. Now I was given a prescription for the same antidepressants I had been on before; at last I felt I was doing something to aid my recovery even though I knew it would take several weeks before I felt the benefit of my medication. I felt even more pleased when the doctor told me to make another appointment for the following Wednesday – at last someone was taking an interest in my case. When I saw the doctor again a week later and started to tell her how I was feeling she said that she really wanted to see me to make sure I was still taking the pills. As I left her surgery she handed me a leaflet and added that if I wanted to talk to her again I could ring the surgery. So, the following week I rang the surgery only to learn that that particular doctor was on leave!

I was beginning to think help was not available but when I read the leaflet the doctor had given me I realised it was about mental health self-referral. I rang the number and was told I could have an appointment in a few weeks. I could not wait weeks, I was beginning to have thoughts of helping myself out of my hell. When I related a bit about my history and stressed how urgent I felt it was, I was given an appointment within a few days. In the meantime I rang the psychologist I had seen in London and we had a couple of sessions on the telephone. Whilst it was lovely to hear her voice again I still didn't feel that I was on my way to recovery. I kept my self-referral appointment and it was a relief to meet someone I could talk to and who had a plan for me. I was to keep a journal and write every day, recording my moods, my activities and thoughts.

Whilst I could write a story or an essay the idea of keeping a journal never really appealed and I found it difficult to write all my thoughts and feelings down on paper. Even so I did my best and returned for my appointment the following week. I desperately clung to the hope that this cognitive behaviour therapy would help me but it seemed a vain hope; nothing had changed yet and I still had thoughts of taking my own opportunity. My symptoms were overriding my heart and dominating my head and the chest pain had now returned with a vengeance, often threatening to consume me with fire. "What can I do?" I asked myself over and over until the answer seemed to come from my own head: "Take your opportunity".

Soon after this, in October, I had an appointment at my hair clinic in London. "Is the train coming in?" asked Colin as we sat on a seat on the platform, looking over his shoulder. I replied, "Yes." He rose from the seat and walked a few steps away from me. I rose from the seat and stared at the train: "Take your opportunity". Of course, this was it.

The next thing I knew I was being dragged along under the train until it finally came to a halt. It seemed very noisy and I could see faces around me of police and medics. I had a few more seconds of awareness thinking it was amazing that I seemed unscathed apart from my ankle, which was trapped under the metal wheel of the train before I was aware of my coat sleeve being cut up my arm and thought oh no! Not my coat! Before I lost consciousness.

Later that day I awoke from surgery to find myself in St George's Hospital, Tooting, London. My foot had been amputated and the surgeon was explaining that I would have to undergo further surgery in a few days to remove more of my leg in order to have the best opportunity for a prosthetic leg. I did not like the idea of losing more of my leg but didn't feel in a position to argue. Somehow I felt absolutely sure that I would walk again anyway.

Late at night two weeks later I was transferred to the Royal Surrey Hospital in Guildford. Now it was much easier for Colin and friends to visit me but unfortunately I was in a geriatric ward and my four weeks in this hospital was not a happy experience. The first thing I heard on my first morning was my neighbouring patient asking why she was still alive, why hadn't she died in the night like she wanted to. I was certainly not feeling suicidal but I was still very anxious and worried about everything; this was not a good environment for me.

I had a gruelling schedule of having to rise early and be ready for hospital transport three times a week to visit Queen Mary's Hospital at Roehampton. I still felt in shock and was recovering from my surgery, I was not sleeping well and still felt very anxious and panicky but in the absence of sufficient in-house physiotherapy I was very grateful for the expertise of the wonderful staff at Queen Mary's. It was progress in the right direction towards getting my prosthetic leg, and the mood in the gym was so positive it helped me greatly.

I desperately wanted to feel better and rid myself of constant anxiety. I tried to be cheered by regular comments and texts from friends with messages of faith in my ability to overcome and win through. I struggled to agree and scared myself with an element of self-doubt. Yes. I had done it before but could I do it again?

After four weeks I was transferred to Farnham Road Hospital in Guildford. A move I had dreaded and for me justifiably. It was a complete culture shock not being allowed to have my phone or tablet charger, a belt to my dressing gown, a manicure set or scissors, etc. Each patient had their own room with sloping window sills, grab rails that were filled in at the back, no plug in the basin and an observation window in the door; everything possible to prevent self-harm. I may not have been in a fully stable state of mind but I certainly had no intention of harming myself and I found the whole set-up abhorrent.

I believed this hospital would provide counselling or talking therapy for me but instead I was observed at regular intervals every twenty-four hours. This meant someone standing by the table with a notepad during meals to write down exactly what was eaten and dark silhouettes at the window in my bedroom or the door being opened throughout the night to check on me. Not being able to walk I was acutely aware of my dependence on staff, especially when using the bathroom for any reason. I felt as though I had completely lost my dignity and privacy – even with one leg and one arm I was still capable of pulling my own pants down and up again! I will never understand why mental health patients are not given the same respect as other patients when it is so vital for their well-being.

I still worried about being ready for my hospital transport and panicked if it was late but at least I still had three visits a week to Roehampton where things were progressing very well. On the way home I used to pray for a traffic jam on the A3 to prevent arriving back early but it never happened. I wanted to spend as little time as possible in the hospital. I could have gone out in the grounds or even been pushed in a wheelchair to the town but I was far too scared to leave the premises once I was inside.

Many friends visited me multiple times and many cards were received. Once again I was overwhelmed by the love and support from friends and family, especially Colin who came every day. At the time I felt guilty, ashamed and unworthy, especially when my friend Kelly turned up. She was my fellow patient friend from The Royal London Hospital more than eight years earlier. She had flown from Gibraltar, where she was on holiday, booked into a Guildford hotel and visited me two days running. It not only took my breath away, I felt very humble and undeserving when she gave me various goodies she had thoughtfully bought for me, especially two beautifully boxed white chocolate angel wings. I felt that if I didn't get better I would be letting everyone down so I tried really hard, concentrating on my exercise routine and thinking in terms of 'little steps'. Eventually it started to work and instead of panicking and worrying I started to look forward and overcome the guilt and shame I felt.

After several weeks attending the gym at Queen Mary's and practising walking with a PAMAid, measurements were taken, computerised imagery was studied, a cast was made and, finally, I had a fitting. Fortunately my cast fitted comfortably and very soon I had a prosthetic leg. Now, I thought, the hard work really starts as I stood upright and held on to the parallel bars in the gym. Needless to say a huge feeling of elation swept over me, soon overtaken by a massive feeling of achievement as I started to walk up and down, then leaving the confines of the parallel bars to wander freely around the gym; it was much easier than I thought.

Christmas was rapidly approaching and my request to go home for the holiday was dependent on me being able to manage the steps at our front door and cope at home so a home visit was arranged. Accompanied by a Physiotherapist and an Occupational Therapist I stepped out of the car, walked across the gravel drive and up the steps to our front door. Colin greeted me in the hall with amazed disbelief. We hugged and wept with joy. It was fantastic and seemed unbelievable after all that had happened and all we had been through. I knew I would walk again and I did.

The joy of being at home with my family for Christmas far outweighed the lack of decorations, gifts and roast turkey. My amazing daughter provided a wonderful roast chicken dinner and enough flowers to decorate several rooms in our flat. It was a wonderful day and my grandchildren aged four and six were too preoccupied by their presents to notice that nanna had a prosthetic leg.

I had to return to hospital for one night as early morning transport was arranged for Queen Mary's Hospital the next day. At a meeting with the Consultant Psychiatrist I told him that if I stayed any longer it would be counter-productive for me. That was my last night in the hospital, only returning a week or so later for my official discharge meeting.

For several weeks I stayed indoors and it was so good to have friends visiting in my own home. Wonderful as this was I knew I had to face the challenge of going out and face the people of Godalming. It seemed quite a hurdle to overcome; I thought everyone would be looking at me knowing what I had done. What about the air ambulance? What about the Katie Piper Foundation? What about my book? What about the choir, keep fit class and swimming club? What about my life? How was I going to face up to it all? Whoa, slow down, Lin, one thing at a time.

One afternoon Colin drove us to Godalming as I wanted to get some "Thank you" cards. As we came out of the shop I noticed a sale across the road in one of my favourite shops. Soon we were crossing the road to have a look in the store. Were people staring at me? No! Even if they were, the joy of being able to walk down the street and enter a shop of my choice far outweighed any embarrassment I might have experienced. I felt I had broken the ice; I could now start to move on with my life. Choir was first after Christmas then keep-fit and then meeting up with friends for lunch or coffee. As soon as I can have a 'shower leg' I want to rejoin the Friday Swimmers Club at Guildford Spectrum.

I will not risk coming off medication again so I am content to take my pills daily as prescribed. Follow-up appointments with a psychiatrist followed my hospital discharge. As I met all the criteria I had the option to have further one-to-one or group therapy. I really felt as though I did not need it but could not deny my past and having got this far I decided to go ahead even though it would mean weekly visits to the hospital for more than a year. I would hate to have future regrets for not taking this opportunity. Nevertheless there is a six month waiting list and in the meantime I have regular visits at home from a lovely Chinese lady psychiatrist. I appreciate all this attention now but wonder why oh why was it not so readily available when I really needed it?

My enthusiasm for life had returned but I still had a feeling that I had messed up and ruined everything. Then one day I had a phone call from John Luff, a man I met and chatted to about a year ago at a local rural life museum. He was editor of the residents' magazine in his area and wanted to publish articles about memorable people he had met. I was first on his list and he wanted to publish my story, even after I told him what had since happened to me. I edited my story to a suitable length, and it went into print.

A month or so later a friend at choir asked if I could help as her local church group needed a speaker at fairly short notice. My talk was to briefly include my story whilst focusing on the work of the Kent Surrey and Sussex Air Ambulance. What a perfect opportunity for my first step back into public speaking.

When we had a phone call from a lady called Caroline from Buckingham Palace we were very wary. It was not a wind-up, despite our doubts – apparently the Kent Surrey and Sussex Air Ambulance had put our names forward and we had been selected to attend one of the Queen's Garden Parties at Buckingham Palace. In due course the official invitation arrived and Colin and I spent a glorious sunny afternoon in the Palace garden, enjoying a yummy tea and meeting some very interesting people. We saw Her Majesty the Queen and His Highness The Duke of Edinburgh and I wandered all over the lawns amid the huge crowd until I finally got my photograph of the royal couple.

I had an email from the amazing young man called Junior Smart who was a fellow speaker at the Samaritans Conference I had attended a couple of years previously. He had been teaching at Greenwich University and had spoken to a tutor about me and now he wanted to introduce her to me. The result was that I appeared on the students' timetable as a tutor and attended for a two hours session one Tuesday afternoon.

Who would have thought that my life would again rise to such a high? I remember a time when I was concerned about what other people thought of me, I know what I think of myself and that is what really matters. I have honesty, integrity, compassion, loyalty, tenacity and time. I have a family I truly love, friendships I truly value and a delight in the joy of living. All enhanced by the knowledge that somewhere along the way I may have helped someone come to terms with understanding a life changing event that has happened to them. Life has returned to normal for me and I have rediscovered my true self. Once again I feel a desire to 'pay back' and hope that somewhere someone can be helped by my story. I feel I am now at a point where I am in control and everything is normal. I intend to maintain the status quo because it must never happen again. Would I ever be that lucky again?

---o0o---